Law and Professional Issues in Midwifery

Richard Griffith,
Cassam Tengnah
and Chantal Patel

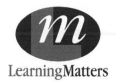
LearningMatters

First published in 2010 by Learning Matters Ltd

British Library Cataloguing in Publication Data
A CIP record for this book is available from the British Library

ISBN: 978 1 84445 469 3

This book is also available in the following ebook formats:

Adobe ebook   ISBN: 978 1 84445 703 8
EPUB ebook   ISBN: 978 1 84445 702 1
Kindle   ISBN: 978 1 84445 992 6

Cover design by Topics – The Creative Partnership
Project Management by Diana Chambers
Typeset by Kelly Winter
Printed and bound in Great Britain by TJ International Ltd, Padstow, Cornwall

Learning Matters Ltd
33 Southernhay East
Exeter EX1 1NX
Tel: 01392 215560
E-mail: info@learningmatters.co.uk
www.learningmatters.co.uk

FSC
Mixed Sources
Product group from well-managed
forests and other controlled sources
Cert no. SGS-COC-2482
www.fsc.org
© 1996 Forest Stewardship Council

Contents

About the authors

Richard Griffith is a lecturer and the law team coordinator at the School of Health Science, Swansea University, where he has taught since 1992. He teaches a wide range of students including midwifery students. He initially trained as a nurse before turning his attention to law and an academic career. He has a particular interest in applied law in nursing practice and has published widely in a range of nursing journals.

Cassam Tengnah is a lecturer in health law at the School of Health Science, Swansea University, and teaches across a range of courses from undergraduate to postgraduate level, including midwifery students. His background is in nursing and health promotion, and he has a particular interest in public health law.

Chantal Patel is a lecturer in health law and ethics at the School of Health Science, Swansea University. Chantal has a wide and varied legal background, and has a particular interest in diversity and the law. Chantal sits as a Justice of the Peace in Swansea.

Acknowledgements

The authors and publishers would like to thank particularly Moira McLean, Senior Lecturer in Midwifery, Supervisor of Midwives, Deputy Lead Midwife and Programme Leader for BSc (Hons) Midwifery at de Montfort University, for her extremely helpful feedback on this book during its development.

We would also like to thank the following reviewers of the proposal and draft material for their helpful suggestions:

Ann Kingscott, Senior Academic, Lead Midwife for Education, Supervisor of Midwives and Programme Leader, Birmingham City University;

Enid Egginton, Senior Lecturer in Midwifery, Birmingham City University;

Annie Rimmer, Senior Lecturer in Midwifery, University of Brighton;

Elinor Clarke, Principal Lecturer, Coventry University;

Julie Hadley, Senior Lecturer in Midwifery, University of Staffordshire.

Table of cases

Introduction

Midwifery practice is underpinned by the law. It is essential that, when registered midwives provide care and treatment to women, they do so in accordance with the law and their professional obligations. Midwives cannot practise in ignorance of the law. Obstetrics and midwifery remain high-risk and litigious areas of healthcare. Over £3.5 billion in compensation has been paid to victims of clinical negligence in obstetrics and midwifery since the NHS clinical negligence scheme began in 1995. This level of financial liability means that maternity services and the midwives who work in them come under increasing scrutiny to ensure that their care and treatment is lawful, professional and ethically justified.

The Nursing and Midwifery Council (NMC) has well-established standards of competence and conduct that must be achieved by all student midwives. These standards are considered the minimum necessary for safe and effective practice. This book is structured so that it will help you to understand and meet the competencies relating to the legal and professional duties that are required for entry to the NMC register as a registered midwife. The relevant competencies from the *Standards for Pre-registration Midwifery Education* (NMC, 2009e) are presented at the start of each chapter so that you can clearly see which ones the chapters address.

Chapter 1 provides you with the essential building blocks for understanding where laws come from, how they develop through cases that come before the courts, and how to locate, read and interpret the different types of law that affect your future role as a registered midwife. By reading closely and completing the activities in this chapter, you will begin to develop a legal awareness that will underpin your midwifery education.

Chapter 2 points out that, during the course of your practice, you will find that you come across situations that give rise to complex dilemmas for which the law does not always provide an easy answer. These situations give rise to questions about whether your actions are morally acceptable and ethically right. This chapter explores the notion of morals in relation to midwifery practice and sets out a framework for a principle-based approach to ethical decision making in the course of your practice as a midwife. The activities in this chapter will help you develop a principled approach to resolving the dilemmas and ensure that you act ethically and in accordance with the law and professional codes of practice.

Chapter 3 draws together the legal and ethical principles introduced in the first two chapters and highlights that, from your first day as a student midwife and throughout you career as a registered midwife, you are accountable for what you do and what you fail to do. The concept of accountability is considered in the context of midwifery. The four spheres of accountability and the standards of conduct they impose through the law are introduced and you will look in some detail at the role of the profession's regulatory body, the NMC, in maintaining public confidence in registered midwives. Understanding accountability is essential for student midwives, who must demonstrate their fitness to practise in order to become registered. As a student you will be subject to the NMC's *Guidance on Professional Conduct for Nursing and Midwifery Students* (2009c).

Chapter 4 explores the notion of rights as they apply to midwifery and focuses in particular on the notion of human rights and the provisions and key concepts of the Human Rights Act 1998. The chapter then discusses how the UK government has had to introduce stronger laws to promote equality and protect people from discrimination. As student midwives you must ensure that your practice respects the rights of the women and babies in your care and you must recognise the needs of the diverse cultures that make up the population of the UK. This chapter emphasises the duty of registered midwives to ensure that they do not discriminate on the grounds of any protected characteristic, such as race or disability, when caring for women.

The rights of women are particularly relevant when considering consent to examination and treatment. Respect for the moral principle of autonomy is essential when making decisions about the examination, care and treatment of a woman, and respect for autonomy is further enhanced by the provisions of the Human Rights Act 1998. Chapter 5 draws together the moral principle of autonomy and the right to respect for a private and family life under human rights law and examines the legal expression of those rights and principles through the law of consent. The chapter considers specific issues, such as free birthing and the refusal of caesarean sections, before taking you through the process of obtaining consent. In this chapter you are also introduced to the concept of decision-making capacity and how the provisions of the Mental Capacity Act 2005 set out the requirements for assessing capacity and making decisions for those women who are unable to make care and treatment decisions for themselves.

Chapter 6 builds on the previous chapter by examining the law of consent as it applies to babies and to mothers who are under 18 years old. It highlights how a minor moves through three developmental stages on the path to becoming an autonomous adult and how infants and young children rely on a person with parental responsibility to consent to examination and treatment on their behalf. The chapter then considers how a midwife would assess the competence of a mother who is under 16 to consent, using the rule in *Gillick*, and the rights of young mothers aged 16 and 17 to consent to treatment. The chapter discusses common dilemmas faced by midwives, such as when a parent disagrees with what treatment their baby should receive or where a young mother refuses to stay in hospital to have treatment.

Chapter 7 continues to consider the rights of children by examining the role of midwives in safeguarding children at risk of significant harm. As a midwife you will have a key role in the identification of infants and children who may have been abused or who are at risk of abuse. You will also be well placed to recognise when parents or other adults have problems that might affect their capacity to fulfil their roles with infants and children safely. It is vital, therefore, that you develop a sound working knowledge of the Children Acts of 1989 and 2004 and know when to make a referral for help when you are in contact with a 'child in need', and how to act on concerns that an infant or child is at risk of significant harm through abuse or neglect.

Chapter 8 discusses why record keeping is a fundamental skill that must be developed to a consistently high standard by student midwives. The chapter emphasises the importance of accurate record keeping in the safety of women and babies and its role in protecting midwives from litigation. By drawing on case law, the chapter highlights the consequences for you of failing to meet the required standards.

Chapter 9 examines why maintaining the confidentiality of a woman's health information is a fundamental element of professional conduct for all registered midwives and a key standard imposed on student midwives by the NMC through their student guide to professional conduct. The chapter considers the scope and sources of a midwife's duty of confidentiality before discussing the circumstances that would allow you to disclose information relating to a woman or her baby. The dilemma you face is that the duty of confidentiality is not absolute and there are exceptions to the rule. It is essential that, as a student midwife, you learn when the general requirement to maintain the confidentiality of a woman's health information can be overridden and information can be properly disclosed to another.

Chapter 10 considers how the law imposes a duty on you to be careful when providing care and treatment to women and their babies through the law of negligence. You will consider the extent of a midwife's duty of care towards women and their babies and why it is essential for you to provide care and treatment that is evidence-based and research-driven in order to meet your legal duty. The chapter concludes with negligence as a criminal act and the likely consequences if your carelessness results in the death of a woman or her baby.

Chapter 11 builds on the general human rights principles considered in Chapter 4 by examining how the law is used to protect vulnerable women from abuse. It begins by defining a vulnerable woman and then considers what is meant by abuse and the forms it may take. The chapter then discusses the powers available to health and social care authorities to protect vulnerable women from harm.

Chapter 12 looks at how assisted conception and the status of an unborn child is regulated by the law. It introduces you to the regulation of treatments to terminate pregnancy and assist couples to conceive, then examines the rules governing parenthood under the Human Fertilisation and Embryology Act 2008. The chapter also discusses the role of the midwife in ensuring that a baby's birth is notified and registered, and outlines what action should be taken when a baby is stillborn or dies shortly after birth.

Chapter 13 considers the law regulating midwives' use of medicines in the course of their practice. Using case law it examines why it is necessary to regulate the use of medicines and discusses the various methods by which a midwife can lawfully supply and administer medicines to a woman and her baby. In particular, the chapter discusses how a midwife is given an exemption from the need for a prescription to supply and administer a range of medicines commonly used in practice.

From the very outset of your midwifery education, your safety and the safety of the women and babies in your care will be of paramount concern to your university and clinical practice area. Chapter 14 explains how they have obligations under the law to protect your health and safety, and how you have a duty to look after your own health and safety and that of the women and babies you care for. You must be able to apply in practice the legal duties imposed by the Health and Safety at Work etc. Act 1974 and its regulations, and this chapter examines the law in relation to midwifery practice. You will be introduced to the key regulations that impose a duty on you to protect the health and safety of the women and babies in your care and the consequences for you if you fail in that duty.

Throughout the book you will find activities that will help you to make sense of, and learn about, the material being presented. Some activities ask you to reflect on aspects of practice, or your experience of it, or the people or situations you encounter. *Reflection* is an essential skill in midwifery, and it helps you to understand the world around you and often to identify how things might be improved.

Other activities will help you develop key skills such as your ability to *think critically* about a topic in order to challenge received wisdom, or your ability to *research a topic and find appropriate information and evidence*, and to be able to make decisions using that evidence in situations that are often difficult and time-pressured. All the activities require you to take a break from reading the text, think through the issues presented and carry out some independent study, possibly using the internet. Where appropriate, there are sample answers presented at the end of each chapter, and these will help you to understand more fully your own reflections and independent study. Remember, academic study will always require independent work; attending lectures will never be enough to be successful on your programme, and these activities will help to deepen your knowledge and understanding of the issues under scrutiny and give you practice at working on your own.

You might want to think about completing the activities as part of your personal development plan (PDP) or portfolio. After completing each activity, write it up in your PDP or portfolio in a section devoted to that particular skill, then look back over time to see how far you have developed. You can also do more of the activities for a key skill that you have identified a weakness in, which will help your skill and confidence in this area.

Chapter 1

Introduction to the law and the legal system

NMC Standards for Pre-registration Midwifery Education

This chapter will address the following competency:

Domain: Professional and ethical practice
- Practise in accordance with relevant legislation. This will include:
  - demonstrating knowledge of legislation relating to health and social policy relevant to midwifery practice.

Chapter aims

After reading this chapter, you will be able to:

- define the term 'law';
- describe the primary and secondary sources of legal material relevant to midwifery practice;
- explain the system of precedent that underpins the common law;
- outline the relevance of law to healthcare;
- identify the benefits of legal awareness to a student midwife.

Introduction

The influence of the law on midwifery practice is examined in this chapter. It begins by highlighting that the Nursing and Midwifery Council's *Code: Standards of conduct, performance and ethics for nurses and midwives* (NMC, 2008a) (known simply as *The Code*), which sets out the standards for professional practice, is underpinned by the law. The chapter then defines the term 'law' and considers how laws are made. The sources of law are then introduced and you are encouraged to become familiar with the key features of an Act of Parliament, a Statutory Instrument and a Case Report. Finally, the chapter highlights the benefits of legal awareness to a student midwife.

Law is fundamental to the study of midwifery. It informs your practice and underpins your relationship with the profession, and with the mothers and babies in your care. It is essential to understand and be able to critically reflect on the legal issues affecting your practice.

When you take on the care of a woman, you undertake a legal duty of care not to harm her or her baby in accordance with the law of negligence. The care and treatment you provide will be based on the law of consent: the informed and freely given permission of the woman will be a prerequisite to any lawful treatment. The legal principle of confidentiality will regulate your ability to disclose information about mothers and babies while they are in your care.

The accountable midwife

As a registered midwife you will be legally and professionally accountable for your actions, irrespective of whether you are following the instruction of another or acting on your own initiative. Healthcare litigation is growing and patients are increasingly prepared to assert their legal rights. Compensation payment in the National Health Service (NHS) is currently running at some £807 million pounds a year, with the total value of reported claims for obstetrics and gynaecology since 1995 now standing at over £3.5 billion (NHSLA, 2009).

It is little wonder, therefore, that the regulatory body for midwives, the Nursing and Midwifery Council (NMC), insists that student midwives practise in accordance within an ethical and legal framework, putting the interests of mothers and babies first.

A thorough and critical appreciation of the legal and professional issues affecting midwifery practice is essential for developing the awareness necessary to satisfy the NMC that you are an accountable practitioner, competent to practise as a registered midwife.

Defining law

Activity 1.1   *Reflection*

Before reading on, think about the laws you are aware of and what their roles are. Write down what you believe the term 'law' means.

Read on for an answer to this activity.

A typical dictionary would define 'law' as:

a rule enacted or customary in a community and recognised as commanding or forbidding certain actions', or 'a body of such rules'.

A key characteristic of law is that it is perceived as binding upon the community. The English word 'law' is derived from Old Norse *lagu* meaning laid down or fixed. The definition suggests that the law is made up of rules, but do all rules have legal force?

Activity 1.2   *Critical thinking*

Consider the following rules. Which do you think are laws?

- Honour your mother and father.
- Do not steal.

Activity 1.2 continued

- Be truthful in all circumstances.
- Do not kill other people.
- Rescue your neighbour's drowning child.
- Register the birth of a child.
- Do not park on double yellow lines.

Read on for an answer to this activity.

Positive rules

Positive rules impose a legal obligation to do or refrain from doing something. If a positive rule is breached a sanction may be imposed for breaking the law.

Normative rules

Normative rules set out what a person should do, or what they should refrain from doing. The word *should* means that the individual is not compelled to abide by normative rules, they simply ought to. Normative rules are based on values that highlight a desired form of conduct, but such rules do not carry legal force.

In Activity 1.2, the positive rules were:

- Do not kill other people: it is a common law offence, the offence of murder, to kill other people.
- Do not park on double yellow lines: parking on double yellow lines constitutes a road traffic offence.
- Do not steal: stealing is an offence under the Theft Act 1968.
- Register the birth of a child: this is an example of the law requiring a particular action, in this case under the Birth and Deaths Registration Act 1874.

The normative rules were:

- Honour your mother and father: this is established through religious teachings and reflects the fifth of the Ten Commandments. It is not a requirement of the law in the UK.
- Be truthful in all circumstances: veracity is a moral or ethical issue – the need to be truthful in law occurs in specific circumstances such as when giving evidence under oath.
- Rescue your neighbour's drowning child: there is generally no duty of simple rescue in the UK. If you had a professional duty (as a lifeguard at a swimming pool, for example) you would be legally obliged to rescue the child.

In some cases the law requires a person to take action (e.g. the requirement to register a birth). More often, the law requires a person to refrain from doing something, such as killing others, parking on double yellow lines or stealing.

Relevance to midwifery

In midwifery practice, normative and positive rules are drawn together. The law imposes a minimum standard of acceptable care and behaviour on you as a registered midwife.

Mothers and babies deserve the best possible care and concern, so your employer and the profession through *The Code* (NMC, 2008a) set standards that are higher than the law expects.

The Code is underpinned by a shared set of values common to all United Kingdom (UK) Healthcare Regulatory Bodies. In a drawing together of both normative and positive rules, it requires that, as a registered midwife, you:

- respect a woman as an individual;
- obtain consent before you give any treatment or care;
- protect confidential information;
- cooperate with others in your team;
- maintain your professional knowledge and competence;
- be trustworthy;
- act to identify and minimise risk to mothers and their babies.

During your training as a student midwife you will be expected to live up to the standards of the NMC's *Code* and the law that underpins them.

Criminal and civil law

The same unlawful action can be dealt with in different ways by the law. For example, touching a person without permission (i.e. without consent) can be both a crime and a tort (the term used to describe a civil wrong). The crime could be charged under the Offences Against the Person Act 1861. This very old statute is still much in force today and forbids many forms of unlawful touching, including actual bodily harm (s47), wounding (ss18 and 20), and even procuring a miscarriage (s58). A crime is an act that is capable of being followed by criminal proceedings and with an outcome, an acquittal or a conviction that is criminal in nature. For example, a black midwife was fined £250 after being convicted by a jury of racially aggravated assault on a white security guard she referred to as 'white trash' (*Manchester Evening News*, 2003).

Unlawful touching can also be pursued through the civil courts as the tort of trespass to the person. The law of tort is primarily concerned with providing a remedy, by way of compensation, to persons who have been harmed by the conduct of others. For example, a woman received £8,000 damages when surgeons performed a sterilisation without her consent (*Devi v West Midlands RHA* [1981]).

The nature of law

From the discussion so far we can define law as:

A rule of human conduct imposed upon and enforced among, the members of a given state.

There are two principles that underpin this notion of law:

- **order**, in the sense that there is a method or system to the creation and implementation of the law; and
- **compulsion**, or the enforcement of obedience to the rules that are laid down by the law.

Sources of law

When studying the law as it applies to midwifery, you will use a range of primary and secondary sources to inform your practice. See Figure 1.1 for more information.

Primary sources of law

Although there are textbooks and periodicals that discuss legal issues in midwifery, whenever possible it is best to study the primary source of law as well. It is better to read for yourself the judgment from the court or a section of an Act of Parliament that affects your practice. This will give you a more detailed understanding.

There are three primary sources of legal material as follows.

- **Legislation**
  - Acts of Parliament, which may also be referred to as statute law or *lex scripta* (written law).
  - Secondary legislation:
    - Statutory Instruments, which are also known as delegated legislation and subordinate legislation.
- **Judicial decisions**
  - These are decisions from cases decided in court, and are also known as the common law or *lex non scripta* (unwritten law from judges).
- **European Community and human rights law**
  - Parliament has allowed these areas to be sources of law by incorporating them through Acts of Parliament (The European Community Act 1972 and the Human Rights Act 1998).

Figure 1.1: Sources of legal material

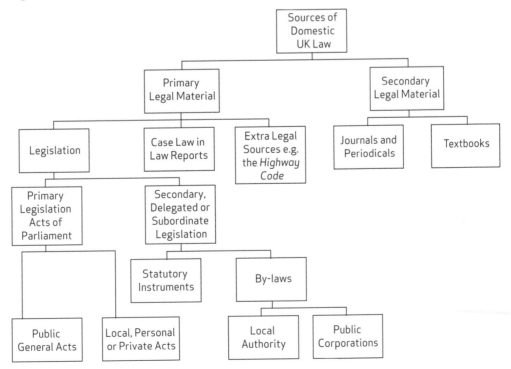

The legal system of the UK goes back many centuries and there is a historical source of law that occasionally has relevance today.

- **Royal Prerogative**
  - The Royal Prerogative used to be the main source of law before the development of the parliamentary system in the UK. It now describes the powers, handed down direct from monarchs to ministers over many years, that allow governments, among other things, to go to war, regulate the Civil Service, issue passports and grant honours, all without any need for approval from Parliament. As these powers have been handed down over many centuries, new powers cannot be created.

When considering a novel dispute or how to apply an ancient law to a modern situation, judges will often take account of extra legal sources to assist them, such as the following.

- **Received wisdom**
  - Legal writers:
    - The law is extensively analysed and tested by academics and practitioners and judges often resort to such analysis to assist them when having to decide a novel or complex case.
  - Public opinion:
    - In *Gillick v West Norfolk and Wisbech AHA* [1986], a case concerning the lawfulness of giving contraceptive treatment to girls under 16, the House of Lords heard an appeal against a decision relying on a seventeenth-century precedent. Lord Scarman said that, in his opinion, part of the court's function was to reflect public opinion and to bring the law kicking and screaming into the twentieth century.
- **Codes and best practice**
  - Judges will also refer to extra legal sources of law that bring together normative and positive rules and signal best practice in a particular area. For example, where a judge has to decide if a midwife's conduct is acceptable, he or she will refer to the NMC *Code* (2008a). In a road traffic case they will refer to the Highway Code. However, these sources are only persuasive and judges are not bound by them.
- **Laws from other countries**
  - Where an issue arises that has never been considered by the courts, judges may consider how the matter was dealt with by the legal system of other countries. The laws and cases of other jurisdictions can be considered by the court, but again they can only be a source of persuasion and are never binding on the court.

Legislation

The UK is a parliamentary democracy and the laws of the country are created and amended through the Queen in Parliament. That is, a new law, or bill, is considered, debated and scrutinised by the elected House of Commons and appointed House of Lords before receiving Royal Assent and becoming an Act of Parliament.

The Acts you are concerned with in your studies are *public general Acts*. These apply to classes or sub-classes of people. For example, the Children Act 1989 concerns the welfare and care of children.

Private Acts, which will not be of great concern to you as a midwife, have a much narrower application and concern local issues and persons. For example, a private Act of Parliament, the Valerie Mary Hill and Alan Monk (Marriage Enabling) Act 1985, was passed to allow a man to marry his ex-wife's mother (his mother-in-law) – an action originally forbidden by the Marriage Act 1960.

The function of Acts

Generally, Acts of Parliament are created to fulfil one of five main functions:

- revision of substantive rules of law;
- consolidation of Acts;
- codification;
- collection of revenue;
- social legislation.

Revision of substantive rules of law

The laws of the UK need to be kept up to date and Acts are created to modernise existing law to bring it into line with modern society. A body known as the Law Commission keeps the law under review and makes suggestions for reform. However, these are not always acted upon in a timely manner. For example, a Law Commission (1993) report into decision making for incapable adults submitted in 1993 eventually resulted in the Mental Capacity Act 2005.

Consolidation of Acts

Laws build up in a piecemeal fashion over many years and there is often a need to consolidate different parts of a law into one Act of Parliament. For example, the Health and Safety at Work etc. Act 1974 consolidated several other Acts, including the Mines and Quarries Act 1954, the Agriculture (Safety, Health and Welfare Provisions) Act 1956, the Factories Act 1961, the Offices, Shops and Railway Premises Act 1963, The Nuclear Installations Act 1965 and the Mines and Quarries (Tips) Act 1969. Similarly, the Equality Act 2010 consolidates anti-discrimination laws into one single Act, the main provisions of which come into force in autumn 2010.

Codification

Codification means putting a rule of the common law, taken from a case decided by a judge in court, into statute law. Where a decision in a case is considered fundamental or very important, Parliament will codify it by making the rule part of an Act. For example, in *R v Bourne* [1939] a surgeon was acquitted of procuring a miscarriage by abortion when a jury decided that doing so to preserve the mental and physical health of the mother was lawful. When the Abortion Act 1967 was enacted, Parliament codified that decision under section 1(1)(c) of the Act.

Collection of revenue

Taxation is a function of Acts. Each year the government presents its budget to Parliament, allowing the raising of revenue through taxation.

Social legislation

This is a broad category that covers the many facets of running the country. It is the main area of party political differences and the main source of debate in Parliament.

How a bill becomes an Act of Parliament

Manifesto

All political parties have a manifesto, which is their book of intentions presented to the electorate of the actions they will take and the laws they will pass if they become the government. It is these that persuade us to vote for a party.

Not all such intentions become law. When a party takes office, detailed information is supplied by senior civil servants and reforms may be found to be unrealistic or too expensive. Other laws enacted during a government's term of office will be a reaction to an event, such as public outrage, a war or a ruling by the courts. In 1993, scientists proposed resolving the shortage of eggs available for assisted conception techniques such as IVF by using the germ cells from aborted foetuses. The public outcry at this forced the government to prohibit their use by hooking a clause on to the Criminal Justice and Public Order Act 1994, section 156, amending the Human Fertilisation and Embryology Act 1990.

Figure 1.2: Stages of a bill

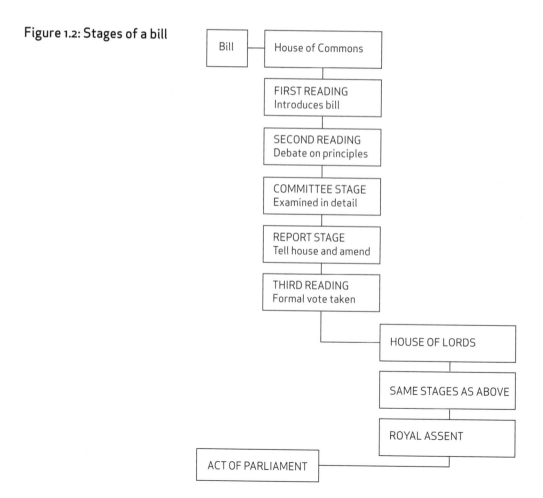

The Queen's Speech

The Queen's Speech at the State Opening of Parliament in November announces the main bills constituting the Government's legislative programme. The government actually writes the speech for the Queen to read.

Green Papers and White Papers

Green Papers (Command Papers) are consultation papers that seek comments from the public. The importance of consultation was seen when Tony Blair attempted to abolish the office of Lord Chancellor without it. He found it to be impossible without first having to change over 500 statutes that referred to functions of the Lord Chancellor.

Following a Green Paper, the Government will often present to Parliament a White Paper, which is a statement of policy and contains definite proposals for legislation. A White Paper may be compared to a brochure advertising the government's intentions and outlining why the change is a positive one.

Bills

In order to become an Act of Parliament, a bill must be passed by both Houses of Parliament and receive Royal Assent (collectively known as 'the Queen in Parliament'). The procedure through which a bill passes to become an Act of Parliament is as follows.

- **First reading**
  The first reading of a bill involves a member reading the title of the bill. This takes place without debate and is essentially an announcement that the bill has been introduced. Copies of the bill are then made available for members to read and are placed on the Parliament website.
- **Second reading**
  The second reading provides the first occasion for debate on the general principles of a bill.
- **Committee stage, House of Commons**
  When a bill has passed its second reading in the House of Commons, it is referred to a General Committee. The Committee examines the clauses of the bill line by line, word by word and detailed amendments are considered.
- **Committee stage, House of Lords**
  In the House of Lords, bills normally go through the committee stage in a committee of the whole House.
- **Report stage**
  Any amendments made during the committee stage must be approved or rejected by the whole House during the report stage. This stage is a detailed debate where further amendments may be made.
- **Third reading**
  The third reading of a bill often follows immediately after the report stage. The bill is reviewed in its final form, including amendments made at earlier stages. Then the final version of the bill is approved and passed by hand – bound in green ribbon – to the Lords. When the Lords return the bill it is bound in red ribbon.

As you can see from Figure 1.2, broadly the same procedure is followed in the House of Lords.

Once all stages have been completed the bill receives Royal Assent and becomes an Act. The date of Royal Assent is not necessarily the date the Act comes into force. Many Acts begin at a later date with the issuing of a commencement order. For example, the

Figure 1.3: The first page of a public general act with its constituent parts labelled

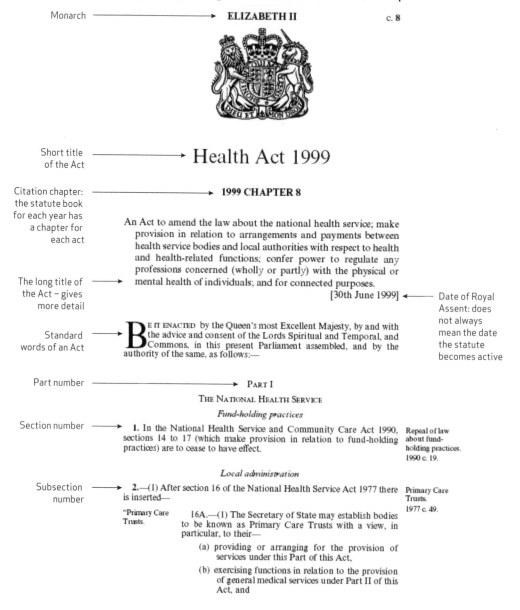

Monarch ⟶ **ELIZABETH II**   c. 8

Short title of the Act ⟶ Health Act 1999

Citation chapter: the statute book for each year has a chapter for each act ⟶ **1999 CHAPTER 8**

An Act to amend the law about the national health service; make provision in relation to arrangements and payments between health service bodies and local authorities with respect to health and health-related functions; confer power to regulate any professions concerned (wholly or partly) with the physical or mental health of individuals; and for connected purposes.

The long title of the Act – gives more detail ⟶

[30th June 1999] ⟵ Date of Royal Assent: does not always mean the date the statute becomes active

Standard words of an Act ⟶ BE IT ENACTED by the Queen's most Excellent Majesty, by and with the advice and consent of the Lords Spiritual and Temporal, and Commons, in this present Parliament assembled, and by the authority of the same, as follows:—

Part number ⟶ PART I

THE NATIONAL HEALTH SERVICE

Fund-holding practices

Section number ⟶ 1. In the National Health Service and Community Care Act 1990, sections 14 to 17 (which make provision in relation to fund-holding practices) are to cease to have effect.   Repeal of law about fund-holding practices. 1990 c. 19.

Local administration

Subsection number ⟶ 2.—(1) After section 16 of the National Health Service Act 1977 there is inserted—   Primary Care Trusts. 1977 c. 49.

"Primary Care Trusts.   16A.—(1) The Secretary of State may establish bodies to be known as Primary Care Trusts with a view, in particular, to their—

(a) providing or arranging for the provision of services under this Part of this Act,

(b) exercising functions in relation to the provision of general medical services under Part II of this Act, and

part of the NHS and Community Care Act 1990 that concerned care in the community did not commence until 1993. The Easter Act 1928, setting Easter Day on a specific date, has never come into force.

Secondary legislation

The rigorous scrutiny that bills undergo means that only about 50 Acts are passed by Parliament each year. To overcome this limitation, it is common for an Act to give powers to government ministers and other public bodies to introduce secondary legislation enabling a general updating of the law. Secondary legislation, also sometimes called subordinate legislation, generally takes the form of Statutory Instruments, which include regulations and orders. For example, the Medicines Act 1968 is over 40 years old but its provisions are kept up to date by ministers using the power they are given under the Act to introduce secondary legislation. The class of person entitled to prescribe medicines was extended by the Medicines for Human Use (Prescribing) (Miscellaneous Amendments) Order 2006 to include midwives (and other health professionals) who met the requirements of the order.

Some 5,000 Statutory Instruments are approved by Parliament each year. An important Statutory Instrument affecting midwifery is the Nursing and Midwifery Order 2001, which established the NMC. The order was created under powers given to ministers by section 60 of the Health Act 1999. The annotated first page of the 2001 Order is shown in Figure 1.4.

Figure 1.4: First page of the Nursing and Midwifery Order 2001, with its constituent parts labelled

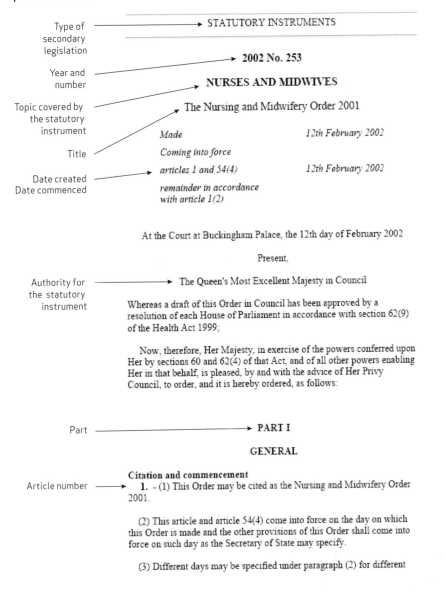

The Nursing and Midwifery Order 2001 established the NMC and gave the organisation powers to regulate and set standards for nurses and midwives. Articles 42 and 43 of this order give the NMC statutory powers to supervise and set standards for midwives. The *Midwives Rules and Standards* (NMC, 2004b) set out these standards, which were approved by Parliament under the Nursing and Midwifery Council (Midwives) Rules Order of Council 2004. The rules impose a legal duty on midwives, for example, to practise in accordance with such standards as the NMC may specify (rule 6), only supply and administer medicines they have been trained to use (rule 10) and keep continuous and detailed records (rule 9). There is a fuller consideration of the *Midwives Rules* in Chapter 3 and specific rules are discussed in detail in the relevant chapters of the book.

If a minister or public body such as the NMC tries to go beyond the powers bestowed on them by an Act of Parliament, the decision can be challenged in court. A good example is *London and Westcliff Properties v Minister of Housing and Local Government* [1961], where a council compulsorily purchased a property, then sold it to a company at reduced cost. The court held that this was *ultra vires* – beyond its powers – as the Housing Act 1957 required councils to obtain the best possible price for a property.

Judicial interpretation of statutes

Once an Act has completed its Parliamentary stages and becomes law, its authoritative and compelling interpretation is for judges and no one else. When it comes to a dispute, only the judges' views count. Governance in the UK is structured to prevent tyranny by attempting to ensure that no one person or body has an over-dominant role. The system sees three components of governance coming together, but as separate entities with different roles as illustrated in Figure 1.5.

Judicial function

The role of the courts is to give force to the intention of Parliament as expressed in the words of an Act and to make decisions between disputing parties. The courts cannot question the validity of statutes as Parliament is supreme: an Act of Parliament is our supreme source of law. Judges must apply the statute to the particular facts before them. To do this they need to interpret the words in an Act.

Parliament makes law. Judges interpret and apply the law and have a great deal of discretion in how they do this.

Figure 1.5: Components of governance in the English legal system

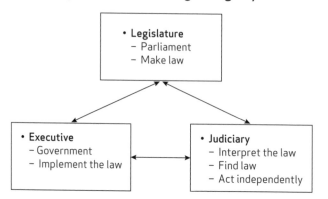

Judicial decisions, the common law

The common law is a body of rules that arise from cases decided by the courts. It works on a system of precedent and is often referred to in Latin as *stare decisis* ('let the decision stand'). A judge considering a case must refer to decisions in previous similar cases in the higher courts and keep to the rulings in those cases. If the previous case was about a similar set of facts and the same legal rules, the current case has to be decided in the same way.

Activity 1.3	Critical thinking

In *Donoghue v Stevenson* [1932] two friends have a drink in a café. Mrs Donoghue has a ginger beer, which she gradually pours from an earthenware bottle and drinks. Eventually, from the bottom of the bottle comes a green sludge, the remains of a decomposing snail. This causes her gastroenteritis and nervous shock, so she sues the manufacturer and the court awards her damages. The court finds that the manufacturer owed her a duty of care, which they have breached, causing her harm because, through their carelessness, a snail entered the bottle in the manufacturing process.

Consider the following situations and decide whether the judge in these cases would be bound by the precedent set in the *Donoghue v Stevenson* [1932] case.

- A woman buys a jar of baby food from a supermarket. Before she opens it she notices a piece of foreign material in the jar. Can she sue in negligence?
- Utilities contractors dig a hole in a pavement and mark it with an upturned sledge hammer. A mother pushing her baby in a pram cannot see the hole, falls in and breaks a leg. Can she sue in negligence?
- A young child is eating fish fingers for school dinner when he chokes on a piece of bone that requires surgery to remove. His mother sues the manufacturers, who say they are not to blame as there is a warning on the package. Are they right?
- A woman has a sterilisation but it is poorly done and she has a healthy child. Can she sue in negligence?

A brief outline answer is given at the end of the chapter.

The structure of the courts

The use of precedent:

- gives certainty to the law;
- prevents arbitrary decisions;
- maintains equality;
- provides a rational basis for decision making.

A court is bound by precedent where the decision of a higher court is materially similar to a case being considered in a lower court. Senior judges ensure that this rule is rigidly enforced.

The courts are structured on a hierarchical system (see Figure 1.6), allowing a series of appeals in the same case.

Figure 1.6: The structure of the courts in England and Wales

United Kingdom Supreme Court
The most senior domestic court
12 members of the Supreme Court sit in benches of up to nine judges
The members are known as Justices of the Supreme Court
Hear Appeals from the Court of Appeal and in exceptional circumstances the High Court

Court of Appeal	
32 Lord Justices of Appeal	
Criminal Division Hears appeals from the Crown Court	**Civil Division** Hears appeals from the High Court, tribunals and certain cases from county courts

The High Court		
92 Justices or Puisne Judges		
Queen's Bench Division Contract and tort Administrative Court Supervises the legality of decisions of inferior courts, tribunals, local authorities, Ministers of the Crown, and other public bodies and officials	**Family Division** Divisional Court Hears appeals from the magistrates' courts	**Chancery Division** Divisional Court Hears appeals from the county courts on bankruptcy and land law

Crown Court Trials of indictable offences, appeals from magistrates' courts, cases for sentence	County Courts Majority of civil litigation subject to nature of the claim

Magistrates' Courts Trials of summary offences, committals to the Crown Court, family proceedings courts and youth courts	Tribunals Hear appeals from decisions on: immigration, social security, child support, pensions, tax and land

It is essential that you, as a student midwife, look carefully at which courts the case has been heard in, and inform your practice by reference to the decision in the most senior court. For example, in *Gillick v West Norfolk and Wisbech AHA* [1986] the case began in the High Court, which decided on the advice to doctors that girls under 16 could be given contraceptive advice, and that treatment without parental consent was lawful if the girl was sufficiently mature and intelligent to make the decision herself. The Court of Appeal overruled the decision of the High Court, declaring the advice unlawful. In the House of Lords, the decision of the Court of Appeal was reversed and the advice declared lawful.

The House of Lords was replaced by the Supreme Court in October 2009 as the most senior court in our judicial system. The justices of the Supreme Court now set out guidance in their opinions that will bind future cases. Opinions in cases from the House of Lords, and the Supreme Court, can be reliably used to inform your practice as a midwife.

To assist with the application of the system of precedent, significant decisions of judges in cases are set out in Law Reports, which lawyers can use to inform their practice. A large number of commercial Law Reports are available, and some cases are even reported in the broadsheet newspapers. Case Reports contain a lot of detail about the facts and law in a case. Many are now freely available from websites of organisations such as the British and Irish Legal Information Institute and they are an excellent source of primary law. Your university law library will have a wide range of Law Reports with cases relevant to midwifery, many of which will be mentioned in this book.

Case law is a particularly relevant source of law in healthcare as the sensitive nature of the disputes inevitably gives rise to decisions that have an impact on how you conduct your midwifery practice.

Devolution in Wales, Scotland and Northern Ireland

Devolution is the granting of powers from the central UK government to the governments of Scotland, Northern Ireland and Wales. Devolved governments were created following referenda in Wales and Scotland, and the Scottish Parliament, National Assembly for Wales and Northern Ireland Assembly were established.

The Scottish Parliament has powers to make primary legislation in certain devolved areas of policy that includes health policy. Law and policy relating to health in Scotland is now for the Scottish Parliament to decide. There are many examples of how health policy in Scotland differs from that in the rest of the UK. For example, the law concerning adults who lack the ability to make decisions comes under the Adults with Incapacity (Scotland) Act 2000 in Scotland but is dealt with under the provisions of the Mental Capacity Act 2005 in England and Wales.

The powers of the National Assembly for Wales and the Northern Ireland Assembly are not as wide ranging as those of the Scottish Parliament. The National Assembly cannot make primary legislation without the approval of the Westminster Parliament, but does have power to make Statutory Instruments that relate to Wales. In Wales, health policy is also a devolved power and, although the primary legislation applies to both England and Wales, the regulations and policy that implement the law differ between the two countries. For example, Wales no longer has prescription charges for medicines, while in England prescription charges continue to rise each year. It is essential to ensure that the policies and laws you apply in your practice relate to the country you work in.

The advantages of legal awareness to a student midwife

The legally aware student midwife:

- **realises that many aspects of daily life are governed by law**
  Most aspects of life are regulated by law. Legal awareness helps you appreciate the importance of the legal framework that supports the structure of society. It also allows you to appreciate that personal and social problems may have a legal dimension.

Figure 1.7: Annotated Law Report

Law report citation

[1994] 1 All ER 819

Title of the case → **Re C (adult: refusal of medical treatment)**

Name of the court → **FAMILY DIVISION**

Name of the judge → **THORPE J**

Dates of the hearing → **8, 11, 14 OCTOBER 1993**

Catchwords →

Medical treatment - Adult patient - Consent to treatment - Right to refuse consent - Mentally ill patient contracting gangrene in leg - Hospital proposing amputation of leg - Patient refusing to consent to amputation - Patient applying for injunction to restrain hospital from amputating leg without his written consent - Whether patient's refusal impaired by mental illness - Whether court should grant injunction - Whether court having jurisdiction to grant injunction restraining future treatment.

Headnote: a summary of the facts and the law in the case →

C, a 68-year-old patient suffering from paranoid schizophrenia, developed gangrene in a foot during his confinement in a secure hospital while serving a seven-year term of imprisonment. He was removed to a general hospital, where the consultant surgeon diagnosed that he was likely to die imminently if the leg was not amputated below the knee. The prognosis was that he had a 15% chance of survival without amputation. C refused to consider amputation. The hospital authorities considered whether the operation could be performed without C's consent and made arrangements for a solicitor to see him concerning his competence to give a reasoned decision. In the meantime, treatment with antibiotics and conservative surgery averted the immediate threat of imminent death but the hospital refused to give an undertaking to the solicitor that in recognition of his repeated refusals it would not amputate in any future circumstances. There was a possibility that C would develop gangrene again. An application was made on C's behalf to the court for an injunction restraining the hospital from carrying out an amputation without his express written consent. On behalf of the hospital it was contended that C's capacity to give a definitive decision had been impaired by his mental illness and that he had failed to appreciate the risk of death if the operation was not performed.

Decision of the court →

Held - The High Court, exercising its inherent jurisdiction, could direct by way of an injunction or declaration that an individual was capable of refusing or consenting to medical treatment, including future medical treatment. However, in determining whether that person had sufficient capacity to refuse treatment, the question to be decided was whether it had been established that his capacity had been so reduced by his chronic mental illness that he did not sufficiently understand the nature, purpose and effects of the proffered medical treatment. That in turn depended on whether he had comprehended and retained information as to the proposed treatment, had believed it and had weighed it in the balance when making a choice. Although C's general capacity to make a decision had been impaired by schizophrenia, the evidence failed to establish that he lacked sufficient understanding of the nature, purpose and effects of the proposed treatment, but instead showed that he had understood and retained the relevant treatment information, believed it and had arrived at a clear choice. It followed that the presumption in favour of his right to self-determination had not been displaced. A declaration would be made accordingly (see p 822 *a* and p 824 *f* to p 825 *a d* to *f*, post).

Figure 1.7 (continued): Annotated Law Report

Re T (Adult: Refusal of Medical Treatment) [1992] 4 All ER 649 and *Airedale NHS Trust v Bland* [1993] 1 All ER 821 applied.

Notes

For consent to medical treatment, see 30 *Halsbury's Laws* (4th edn reissue) para 39, and for cases on the subject, see 33 *Digest* (Reissue) 273-275, *2242-2246*.

Cases referred to in judgment

Airedale NHS Trust v Bland [1993] 1 All ER 821, [1993] AC 789, [1993] 2 WLR 316, HL.   ◄——— Law cases discussed in the judgment

T (adult: refusal of medical treatment), Re [1992] 4 All ER 649, [1993] Fam 95, [1992] 3 WLR 782, CA.

Originating summons

By an originating summons issued on 4 October 1993, C, a patient   ◄——— The lawyers arguing the case
confined to Broadmoor Hospital, sought an injunction retraining the defendants, Heatherwood Hospital, Ascot, from amputating his right leg in the present and future without his express written consent. The summons was heard in chambers but judgment was given by Thrope J in open court. The facts are set out in the judgment.

Richard Gordon and Craig Barlow (instructed by Scott-Moncrieff & Harbour, Brighton) for the plaintiff.

Adrian Hopkins (instructed by J Tickle & Co) for the defendants.
P A B Jackson (instructed by the Official Solicitor) as amicus curiae.

THORPE J.

This originating summons was issued on 4 October 1993 by C. It seeks under the court's inherent jurisdiction an injunction restraining Heatherwood Hospital, Ascot from amputating his right leg without his express written consent.

The plaintiff is 68 and of Jamaican origin. He came to England in 1956, his   ◄——— The judgment of the court in detail
passage being paid by the woman with whom he had lived since 1949. In 1961 she left him, and in 1962 he accosted her at work and after an altercation stabbed her. He was sentenced at the Old Bailey to seven years' imprisonment. While serving that sentence he was diagnosed as mentally ill and transferred from Brixton to Broadmoor. On admission he was diagnosed as suffering from chronic paranoid schizophrenia. He was treated both with drugs and ECT. Over the years he has mellowed and has been accommodated for the past six years on an open ward of the parole house. He is described as neat and tidy, becoming more sociable with staff and other patients in the past two years.

- **knowingly acts in accordance with legal principles**
  Many parts of the law are necessarily complex and difficult to understand. However, the underlying principles are quite simple. These affect everyone on a day-to-day basis, so an understanding of them is important. Ignorance of the law can bring very serious consequences.
- **understands the key elements of the legal system**
  Knowledge of the law is of limited value unless you understand the various ways in which the legal system works to enforce the law. It is important to understand the role of those agencies that have powers to enforce the law and of the mechanisms by which you can seek legal help and advice.
- **knows when and where to seek appropriate advice**
  The law is vast and constantly changing. You need to develop a sense of:
  - when the law can help or hinder;
  - what you can find out for yourself and where;
  - when you should seek expert help;
  - how to get the appropriate help or advice.
- **understands the nature of law**
  Even though many day-to-day situations have a legal dimension, there are some problems that the law can do little about, even when in theory this should not be the case.

C H A P T E R   S U M M A R Y

- A thorough and critical appreciation of the legal and professional issues affecting midwifery practice is essential for developing the awareness necessary to become a registered midwife.
- Positive rules impose a legal obligation to do, or refrain from doing, something. If a positive rule is breached, a sanction may be imposed for breaking the law.
- Normative rules set out what a person should do.
- Midwifery practice sees a drawing together of normative and positive rules.
- Law is defined as a rule of human conduct imposed upon, and enforced among, the members of a given state.
- The UK is a parliamentary democracy and the laws of the country are created and amended through the Queen in Parliament.
- Once an Act has completed its parliamentary stages and becomes law, the authoritative and compelling interpretation of that statute is for judges and no one else.
- An Act of Parliament is our supreme source of law.
- The common law is derived from decided cases and works through a system of precedent that ensures materially similar cases are decided in the same way, thus creating a degree of certainty in the law.

Activities: brief outline answers

Activity 1.3: Critical thinking (page 17)

- The woman in the first case cannot sue in negligence as she has not suffered a personal injury. She discovered the foreign matter before giving her baby the food.
- Although the facts in the second case seem very different, the case is still materially similar to *Donoghue v Stevenson* [1932]. The contractor owes a duty of

care to other users of the footpath, and has failed to take adequate precautions to prevent a fall. It is reasonably foreseeable that the view of the hole may be impaired by an object such as a pram. Harm has been caused by the contractor breaching its duty of care, so a claim in negligence is possible.

- The facts and rules in the third example appear similar but the manufacturer is arguing that the warning absolves them of their duty of care. You might argue, however, that as the fillet fish fingers are marketed towards children, the manufacturer should take greater care. This case was settled out of court with a compensation payment.
- At first glance the fourth example again appears to be a case of carelessness, but to be actionable, as in *Donoghue v Stevenson* [1932], there must be harm to the individual. The courts consider a healthy child as an economic loss not a personal injury. No claim for negligence would succeed for carelessness that resulted in the birth of a healthy baby.

Knowledge review

Having completed the chapter, how would you now rate your knowledge of the following topics?

	Good	Adequate	Poor
1. The primary and secondary sources of legal material.			
2. The role of statutes in law.			
3. The role of precedent in common law.			
4. The benefits of legal awareness to your midwifery education.			
5. Learning to learn.			

Where you're not confident in your knowledge of a topic, what will you do next?

Further reading

To understand the law and how it applies, it is essential to have some knowledge of legal method. One of the following will help:

Hanson, S (2009) *Legal Method, Skills and Reasoning*, 3rd edn. London: Routledge-Cavendish.

Holland, J and Webb, J (2006) *Learning Legal Rules: A student's guide to legal method and reasoning*. London: Blackstone Press.

To understand law in context it is useful to have an understanding of health and maternity policy. The following are recommended:

Crinson, I (2008) *Health Policy: A Critical Perspective*. London: Sage.

Downe, S (ed) (2008) *Normal Childbirth: Evidence and debate*. London: Churchill Livingstone.

Ham, C (2009) *Health Policy in Britain*, 6th edn. London: Palgrave Macmillan.

Mander, R (2007) *Caesarean: Just Another Way of Birth?* London: Routledge.

Useful websites

To keep up to date with changes in health law we recommend:

www.bailii.org British and Irish Legal Information Institute, which provides free access to Law Reports from the UK courts.

www.dh.gov.uk Outlines government policy on health in England.

www.opsi.gov.uk/ legislation/uk.htm Gives full text of legislation and Statutory Instruments.

And for Welsh and Scottish government health policy and publications:

http://wales.gov.uk/topics/health

www.scotland.gov.uk/Topics/Health

Chapter 2

Principled decision making and ethics

NMC Standards for Pre-registration Midwifery Education

This chapter will address the following competencies:

Domain: Professional and ethical practice

- Practise in accordance with relevant legislation. This will include:
  - demonstrating knowledge of contemporary ethical issues and their impact on midwifery practice
  - managing the complexities arising from ethical and legal dilemmas.
- Practise in a way which respects, promotes and supports individuals' rights, interests, preferences, beliefs and cultures.

Chapter aims

After reading this chapter, you will be able to:

- describe the terms 'morals' and 'ethics';
- outline the principle-based approach to decision making;
- identify how the principle-based approach can be used when considering a moral problem relating to practice.

Introduction

The requirement of midwives to practise in a way that is accepted by law and the professional code of conduct (NMC, 2008a) has been discussed in the previous chapter. However, during the course of your practice, you will find that you will come across many situations that give rise to complex dilemmas where the law does not always provide an answer. These situations raise questions about whether an action is morally acceptable and ethically right. This chapter will explore the notion of morals as they apply to midwifery practice. The meaning of 'morals' and 'ethics' will be considered and some of the common dilemmas arising in midwifery practice will be discussed. The chapter then provides a framework for a principle-based approach for use when making decisions in the course of your professional practice.

This chapter and the activities will enable you to develop a principled-based approach to resolving the dilemmas you will encounter as a midwife and ensure that you act in a way that is ethically based and acceptable under the law and your professional code of conduct.

Moral dilemmas in midwifery

You will undoubtedly come across many situations during the course of your day-to-day work where no clear conclusion can be immediately drawn from your understanding of either the law or the professional *Code*. For example, a midwife may believe that a doctor's decision not to resuscitate a severely ill baby with severe birth defects is wrong. The midwife may believe that the sanctity of human life should be respected and that the baby's life should be sustained. The doctor's decision to withhold resuscitation and the midwife's desire to preserve life are both lawful. Neither is proposing to act unlawfully, so the decision is one of morality.

Morals are influenced not only by the law but by culture, religion, beliefs, values, personal conscience, personal convictions and experience. All midwives will find that some clinical decisions are morally acceptable to them, and others are not. To develop an understanding of ethics and morality it is essential that these dilemmas are explored and analysed to provide clarity where there is conflict.

Moral issues and ethical approaches

Before we move on to consider moral issues and how they may be addressed, complete Activity 2.1.

Activity 2.1   *Critical thinking*

A mother, who is totally blind, gave birth to a very premature baby girl. Immediately after the birth, the baby was rushed to the special care baby unit. The mother could not accompany her daughter as she had suffered complications requiring specialist interventions. The baby died within a few hours and the mother was not able to see her baby alive. The mother, although quite ill, was informed of the death. She told the midwife that she would dearly love to hold her baby in her arms for a few minutes.

Two days later, the midwife managed to take her to the mortuary so that she could hold her baby and say goodbye. She was very pleased to have been given the opportunity to spend some time with her first child and was grateful to the midwife.

Later that day, the midwife learnt that there had been a labelling mistake on the coffin and the mother had been given the wrong baby to hold. In the meantime, the mother's condition began to deteriorate rapidly and she started to lapse in and out of consciousness. On one occasion when she was conscious for a few minutes, she thanked the midwife and told her that she felt at peace knowing that she had held, hugged, kissed and said a last goodbye to her baby.

The midwife was upset about what had happened, and was also concerned about whether to tell the mother about the mistake. She knew that, if the mother was told the truth, she would be very upset. On the other hand, she could keep quiet and let the mother live her last moments with the belief that she had been able to hold and say goodbye to her baby.

Activity 2.1 continued

- What would you do in this situation? Write down what you believe should be the decisions made to deal with this situation, and give the reasons for whatever you decide.

The aim of this activity is to allow you to explore what you believe is right or wrong, so there is no outline answer at the end of the chapter.

You probably considered many issues when deciding what you believe to be the right decision and best course of action in this situation. For example, you may believe that the mother has a right to be told the truth, and that telling it is your duty. This belief may be based on factors such as your culture, upbringing, experience, religion or conscience. You may also have considered what would happen if the mother found out that she had not been told the truth. Would she report you to someone in authority? Would disciplinary action be taken against you? Would she lose confidence in you and the midwifery profession?

On the other hand, you may consider that the truth will hurt deeply and for a long time. You may believe that your duty is to protect her from hurt and ensure her happiness and well-being. So you may feel it to be in her best interests not to tell her the truth. At least she will be happy and will have fond memories of being able to hold and say goodbye to her baby.

Many different issues have emerged from the above activity. You have had to judge what you believe is right and, in doing so, you have applied some key ethical principles to this moral conundrum. It is likely that you have at least considered the principles of:

- rights (the right of the mother to be told the truth);
- duty (your duty not to lie to the mother);
- veracity (telling the truth about what has happened);
- consequence (of lying to the mother);
- beneficence (doing good to the mother);
- non-maleficence (doing no harm to the mother).

Activity 2.2   *Reflection*

The examples above are some of the principles that you are likely to have considered when addressing the moral dilemma in Activity 2.1.

- Look again at what you have written and tick any issues that are more or less similar to those highlighted above.

As this activity is based on your own experience and opinions, there is no outline answer at the end of the chapter.

The principles listed above are examples of ethical approaches that may be used to judge the right or wrong of a decision where there is a moral dilemma. The approaches do not provide you with an answer; they enhance your ability to analyse situations and make a decision based on the moral principles underpinning midwifery practice.

Morals and ethics

According to Thompson et al. (2000), morals and ethics are terms used to refer to social customs regarding the rights and wrongs, in theory and practice, of human behaviour. 'Moral' refers to what a person believes is right or wrong based on their culture, experience, upbringing, education, religion, personal convictions and conscience. For example, some people believe that the sanctity of human life should always be respected and that all patients should be treated even if they refuse to give consent. Others may believe that the sanctity of human life should not be respected where it merely prolongs the suffering of an individual, such as a baby born with severe birth defects and in intractable pain. A person's morals are founded on their beliefs and values. Decisions made by that individual will be influenced by those beliefs and values. You will have your own set of beliefs and values – your own moral background that will influence your decisions when caring for a person.

You may think it is morally wrong not to treat a patient who has refused a life-saving blood transfusion. This may well be based on the belief that the sanctity of life should be respected at all times. The decision in allowing the patient and her unborn child to die may be uncomfortable to you. You may want to force your views and beliefs about the sanctity of life on to the patient and doctor. You may even consider ways of forcing the patient to have the blood transfusion. You may consider her children and feel that their wishes should also be respected. You may even consider that the unborn child has a right to life and you have a moral obligation to fight for his or her right. All these are what you believe are the right things to consider and act upon.

However, what you consider to be right could in itself be immoral. It could be argued that the patient has a right to refuse treatment and that her autonomy should be respected. As such, a patient must not be forced to accept treatment just because others believe it is right. Such coercion may be viewed as immoral, unprofessional and unlawful. This gives rise to a moral dilemma which needs to be considered.

A moral dilemma, according to Thompson et al. (2000), is a choice between two equally unsatisfactory alternatives. For example, on the one hand, you may believe that a patient is capable of making a decision to refuse treatment and this should be respected (respect for autonomy). On the other hand, another midwife may believe that one must always act in a way that promotes the well-being of others and decide to treat the woman despite her refusal to consent to that treatment.

This is where ethics and the application of ethical principles will help you to judge the right or wrong of a decision.

Edwards (2009) describes ethics as the enquiry into moral situations and the language employed to describe them. So ethics involves the application of principles to a moral problem in order to help judge if an action is right or wrong.

A principle-based approach to ethical decision making

Beauchamp and Childress (1989) described an approach to the ethics of healthcare that is based on four prima facie moral principles and attention to their application. The four principles approach argues that, whatever our personal philosophy, politics, religion, moral theory or life stance, we will be able to commit ourselves to these four prima facie moral principles. These principles are considered to encompass most of the moral issues that arise in healthcare.

'Prima facie' means that the principle is binding unless it conflicts with another moral principle; if it does, you will have to choose between them. This approach does not provide a method for choosing the right answer to a moral dilemma, but it will provide a common set of moral commitments, a common moral language, and a common set of moral issues (Gillon, 1994).

Beauchamp and Childress's (1989) four moral principles are:

- respect for autonomy, i.e. for the right of a person to decide for him- or herself;
- non-maleficence, which is an obligation not to harm others;
- beneficence, which involves acting in ways that promote the well-being of others;
- justice, which is an obligation to treat others fairly.

Autonomy

The first principle, respect for autonomy, requires respect for the choice made by an individual. In a healthcare context, this means that patients have a right to decide whether or not to undergo any healthcare intervention, even if the refusal will lead to harm or death. The term 'autonomy' is derived from the Greek meaning 'self-governing' and refers to the capacity of an individual to make an informed and uncoerced decision about his or her future. Autonomy is about self-rule with no control, undue influence or interference from others. It respects individuals' choices based on their own values and beliefs.

Gillon (1994) referred to three concepts of autonomy.

- **Autonomy of thought** involves deciding for oneself using all available information and weighing this information.
- **Autonomy of will** involves the intention to do something as a result of a decision.
- **Autonomy of action** involves doing something based on one's decision (e.g. refusing to consent to treatment, like the young mother refusing a blood transfusion in Activity 2.4 above).

Beneficence and non-maleficence

Gillon (1994) argues that, whenever a health professional tries to help others, they inevitably risk harming them. Midwives must therefore consider the principles of beneficence and non-maleficence together with the aim of ensuring benefit to the patient rather than harm.

The NMC *Code* (2008a) underpins a moral and professional obligation to provide overall benefit to patients with minimal harm – that is, beneficence with non-maleficence. To achieve this midwives are committed to a wide range of obligations. Midwives must ensure that they are able to deliver competent, safe care and thus need rigorous and effective education and training both before and during their professional careers. They must also ensure that care is of benefit to the patient. In doing this midwives must respect the patient's autonomy. What constitutes benefit for one patient may be harm for another. For example, a hysterectomy may constitute an overall benefit for one woman with cancer, while for another the destruction of part of her femininity may be so harmful that it cannot be outweighed by the prospect of extended life expectancy.

CASE STUDY: Beneficence and non-maleficence

A popular male midwife who defied hospital rules to help a mother give birth at home was sacked by his employer (*Stamford Mercury*, 2007). The dismissal of the midwife stunned his supporters, who continued to stand by a man they have hailed for risking his career to help women give birth in familiar surroundings. Even his MP tried to table a motion in Parliament to debate the matter. [The midwife] landed himself in hot water after he helped the woman deliver her baby at her home after the Trust had suspended its home birth service due to staff shortages. According to the policy there should be two midwives present at a home birth. He claimed the decision to suspend home birth was financially motivated, a breach of women's rights and a breach of the rules of the Nursing and Midwifery Council. Despite his good intention, he was also held to account by the NMC. A disciplinary panel found that his actions had amounted to misconduct, but chose to caution him rather than strike him off.

Justice

The fourth principle is justice, that is, an obligation to treat others fairly. Justice includes the principles of fairness, equity and an entitlement to what is deserved. Gillon (1994) suggests that the principle can be divided into three categories:

- **distributive justice** – fair distribution of scarce resources;
- **rights-based justice** – respect for people's rights;
- **legal justice** – respect for morally acceptable laws.

Equality is at the heart of justice. In order to achieve fair outcomes for all, it is important to treat equals equally, and those who are not equal in a way that makes good the deficits. In the context of the allocation of resources, conflicts exist between moral concerns such as:

- providing sufficient healthcare to meet the needs of all who need it;
- when this is impossible, distributing healthcare resources in proportion to the need for healthcare;
- allowing midwives to give priority to the needs of their patients;
- providing equal access to healthcare;
- allowing people as much choice as possible in selecting their healthcare;
- respecting the autonomy of those who provide resources by limiting the cost to taxpayers.

All these criteria for allocating healthcare resources can be morally justified but not all can be fully met.

Rights-based justice requires respect for patients' rights. Midwives have no special privilege as health workers to create rights for women or decide which rights should apply. A midwife's disapproval of particular lifestyles will not provide a morally defensible justification for refusing to care for a pregnant woman with AIDS.

The principle of justice requires midwives to obey morally acceptable laws. Even though you may disapprove of the law, you are morally obliged to obey it.

CASE STUDY: Justice

In November 2009, it was reported that pregnant mothers were to be banned from giving birth at their local hospital if midwives considered them to be too fat. The NHS Trust has decided that women with a BMI over 34 would be turned away because of fears among staff that the mothers could die during labour. That triggered a claim that larger women were being unfairly treated because they had to travel miles away to give birth.

Applying the four principles

Activity 2.5   *Critical thinking and group work*

MB, a patient, is 40 weeks pregnant and the baby is in a breech position. She is told that a vaginal delivery would pose serious risks to the child and that a caesarean section will improve the child's chances of survival. She has consented on more than one occasion to the operation but has subsequently withdrawn her consent on each occasion due to her irrational fear of needles. The patient is now in labour. She continues to refuse consent for the injection.

- In a group apply the four principles to this situation and consider if the caesarean should proceed despite MB's objections.

As the answer depends on your own observations, there is no outline answer at the end of the chapter.

Respect for autonomy

This principle entails taking into account and giving consideration to the woman's views on treatment. Autonomy is not an all-or-nothing concept. MB may not be fully autonomous and so not legally competent to refuse treatment, but this does not mean that ethically her views should not be considered and respected as far a possible. She has expressed her wishes clearly: she does not want a needle inserted for the anaesthetic. An autonomous decision does not have to be the correct decision (otherwise individual needs and values would not be respected), but it does have to be informed. Has MB been given information about the consequences of refusing treatment in a manner that she can understand?

Beneficence

Midwives must act to benefit their patients. This principle may clash with the principle of autonomy when a woman makes a decision that is not in her best interests. We must consider both the long-term and short-term effects of overriding MB's views. In the short term, MB will be frightened to have a needle inserted in her arm and to be in hospital; this may lead her to distrust healthcare professionals and be reluctant to seek medical help. In the long-term, there will be a benefit to MB if her autonomy is overridden, as without treatment she will die along with her unborn child.

The benefits of acting in her best interests would need to be weighed against the dis-benefits of failing to respect MB's autonomy. From a legal point of view, the wishes of a competent patient cannot be overridden in their best interests.

Non-maleficence

Non-maleficence means doing no harm to the patient. MB would be harmed by forcibly restraining her in order to insert the needle for anaesthesia, but if she is not treated immediately both she and her child will die.

Which course of action would result in the greatest harm? The assessment relies on assumptions: how successful the operation is likely to be, and how likely it is that MB will be willing and able to care for her child.

Justice

It would be relevant to consider cost-effectiveness of the treatment options for MB, and the impact the decision about her treatment has on her child. However, if she is a competent adult who refuses treatment despite acknowledging the risk to her life and that of her child, you are morally and legally obliged to respect her rights and obey the law. Where there is a conflict between a mother and her unborn child, the law resolves it in favour of the mother. You would have to obey the law even though you may believe that an unborn child should have a right to be born alive.

The principle-based approach concerns autonomy, non-maleficence, beneficence and justice. Using these principles may not necessarily provide you with answers in all situations. Instead, the principles will inform your practice so that you are able to make decisions that are morally justified, professionally recognised and lawful. In the face of any conflict, it is important to remember that you must practise within legal boundaries and professional regulations.

C H A P T E R   S U M M A R Y

- A thorough and critical appreciation of ethical issues affecting midwifery practice is essential if you are to develop the professional awareness necessary to become a registered midwife.
- Many situations in healthcare practice may give rise to questions about whether such practice is morally acceptable and ethically right.
- 'Moral' refers to what we believe is right or wrong and this is based on our culture, experience, upbringing, education and religion.
- 'Ethics' refers to the application of certain principles or theories to a moral problem in order to judge if an action is right or wrong.
- The application of the principles will depend on their relevance to the moral conflicts being judged.
- In the face of any conflict, it is important to remember that you must practise within legal boundaries and professional regulations.

Knowledge review

Having completed the chapter, how would you now rate your knowledge of the following topics?

	Good	Adequate	Poor
1. The terms 'morals' and 'ethics'.			
2. The principle-based approach to healthcare ethics.			
3. How this approach can be used when considering a moral problem relating to practice.			

Where you're not confident in your knowledge of a topic, what will you do next?

Further reading

To further explore the notion of a principle-based approach to decision making. we recommend:
Edwards, SD (2009) *Nursing Ethics*, 2nd edn. Basingstoke: Palgrave Macmillan.

To appreciate the range of dilemmas you are likely to encounter as midwifery students, we recommend:
Journal of Medical Ethics: Journal of the Institute of Medical Ethics. BMJ Publishing.

Useful websites

www.internationalmidwives.org International Confederation of Midwives *Code of Ethics for Midwives.*
The *Code* was originally published in 1993 and updated in 1999 and 2003. It covers midwifery relationships, professional responsibilities of midwives, practice of midwifery and advancement of midwifery knowledge and practice.

www.nmc-uk.org Nursing and Midwifery Council.
You must inform your decision making with up-to-date professional advice and information from the NMC. For advice and guidance on good midwifery practice always refer to *The Code: Standards of conduct, performance and ethics for nurses and midwives.*

Chapter 3

Accountability in midwifery practice

Chapter aims

After reading this chapter, you will be able to:

- define the terms 'accountability' and 'responsibility';
- state the four spheres of accountability in midwifery practice;
- outline the conduct required to avoid liability in each of these four spheres;
- determine whether accountability can be exercised;
- evaluate the role of accountability in midwifery practice.

Introduction

In Chapters 1 and 2, legal and ethical principles were introduced and discussed. This chapter draws these together, highlighting that, from your first day as a student midwife and throughout your career as a registered midwife, you are accountable for what you do and what you fail to do. The chapter begins by considering a definition of the term 'accountability' and how it applies in midwifery. Then the four spheres of accountability and the standards of conduct they impose through the law are introduced. The chapter concludes by looking at the role of the profession's regulatory body, the Nursing and Midwifery Council (NMC), in maintaining public confidence in registered midwives.

The word 'accountability' is familiar to midwives, as it is a term in almost daily use in professional practice. It is included in many midwifery texts and Trust policies and it underpins the NMC's *Code* (2008a). However, despite its common use, the concept of accountability is frequently misunderstood. In a study by Savage and Moore (2004), the term was found to be elusive and ambiguous. Yet accountability is a fundamental concept crucial to the protection of the public and individuals in the care of midwives. It is essential that the term is clearly understood, as it is the means by which the law imposes standards and boundaries on professional practice.

Activity 3.1   *Group work*

In a group, each write down your understanding of the term 'accountability' and how it relates to midwifery practice.

Now read the following for further guidance.

Defining accountability

In their seminal work, Lewis and Batey (1982, p10) defined accountability as:

> *the fulfilment of a formal obligation to disclose to referent others the purposes, principles, procedures, relationships, results, income and expenditures for which one has authority.*

This definition reveals the fundamental nature of accountability. The 'fulfilment of a formal obligation' suggests a basis in law. There is a formal or legal relationship between the midwife and the 'referent others' or higher authorities that hold you to account. The extent of their scrutiny includes 'the purposes, principles, procedures, relationships, results, income and expenditures for which one has authority'. It is not just your conduct but also your competence and integrity that can be called to account.

To be accountable is to be answerable for your acts and omissions. This is the approach adopted by the NMC:

> *You are personally accountable for your practice. This means that you are answerable for your actions and omissions, regardless of advice or directions from another professional.*
>
> (NMC, 2004b)

Accountability or responsibility?

The words accountability and responsibility are often used interchangeably by health-care professionals. Accountability means being answerable to a higher authority for your actions. In contrast, however, responsibility is defined by the *Oxford English Dictionary* as: *Having control or authority over someone or something.*

As a midwife you are responsible for your practice. You decide in what way you practise and what interventions are in the best interests of the women in your care. However, you do not have control or authority over who holds you to account or what you are accountable for. You are required to work within the law and in accordance with the NMC's *Code* (2008a) and the *Midwives Rules and Standards* (NMC, 2004b).

Activity 3.2   *Critical thinking*

The word responsibility is also often used in healthcare.

- Write down your understanding of the word responsibility. Begin by focusing on the general meaning of the word. Then apply this in the context of healthcare.

As this activity is for your own reflection, there is no outline answer at the end of the chapter.

CASE STUDY: *Midwife errors lead to emergency caesarean*

A series of errors by a midwife led to a woman having to undergo an emergency caesarean section. The midwife had failed to properly monitor the high-risk woman and was unable to identify the foetal position of the baby after three internal examinations. She also failed to record the foetal heart rate and maternal pulse every 15 minutes as required by Trust guidelines.

At a fitness to practise hearing the midwife was found to have had a good manner with women, but did not fully understand the width and depth of her sphere of responsibilities.

The NMC hearing concluded that it was clear the midwife was unable to display the skills and abilities required of her. She was struck off the professional register (NMC, 2010a).

Exercising accountability

The NMC (2008a) argues that the purpose of *The Code* is to inform nurses and midwives of the standards of professional conduct required of them in the *exercise of their professional accountability*. Exercising accountability requires the practitioner to have control over what they are accountable for. It suggests that midwives can pick and choose whether they wish to be accountable for this action or that baby. This cannot be the case. The sole purpose of accountability is to protect the public and offer redress to those who have been harmed by your acts or omissions. As a midwife you are answerable to a higher authority: you cannot choose what you are accountable for.

The purpose of accountability

The principle aim of holding midwives accountable for their actions is to ensure that the public and expectant mothers and their babies are not harmed by their acts and omissions, and to provide redress to those who have been harmed. To achieve this, accountability has the following functions.

- A **protective function** to protect the public from the acts or omissions of midwives that might cause harm. You can be called to account for your conduct and competence if it is thought that you have fallen below the standard required of you in law.
- A **deterrent function** as the sanctions available to the authorities hold you to account, and protect the public and patients by discouraging you from acting in a

way that would be considered to be misconduct or unlawful. Registered midwives must act at all times in a manner worthy of a midwife: in work, in public and in their private lives.

- **A regulatory function** making you accountable to a range of higher authorities. The regulatory framework makes it clear what standards of conduct and competence you are required to comply with as a registered midwife.
- **An educative function** as the public scrutiny of a midwife's conduct allows other members of the profession to learn from the mistakes of others. Midwives who are called to account and asked to justify their actions have their cases heard in public with a view to reassuring patients that only the highest standards of practice will be tolerated.

CASE STUDY: Breech birth

A midwife was struck off after mistaking a baby's bottom for his head (*Manchester Evening News*, 2009). She failed to realise that she was dealing with a difficult breech birth despite a scan showing the problem. Although breech presentations can be difficult to diagnose, in this case the baby was presenting feet first, so it was obvious that something was unusual. Despite considerable support from employers and colleagues, her competence did not improve, and she deliberately chose to work on shifts when her mentor was not working. The NMC panel considered her conduct and attitude fundamentally incompatible with continuing to be a registered midwife. She was struck off.

Spheres of accountability

As a midwife you have a formal obligation to answer for your actions to a range of higher authorities that have a legal relationship with you, enabling them to demand that you justify your actions. If you fail to satisfy those requirements, sanctions may be applied against you. For example, during your training, the university and the NHS Trust have legal authority over you. They can hold you to account through reasonable disciplinary measures, or can impose sanctions that could lead to dismissal from your course.

Activity 3.3   *Reflection*

List the authorities that can hold you to account in your role as a midwife. To help you, think of the authorities that offer protection to the public, including the women and babies in your care.

See Figure 3.1 for the answers.

In order to provide maximum protection against misconduct by registered midwives, four areas of law are drawn together and can individually or collectively hold you to account.

Figure 3.1 depicts these four spheres of accountability and highlights the authorities that can hold you to account as a registered midwife. In each case, a legal relationship exists that allows you to be called to account for your actions.

Figure 3.1: Spheres of accountability

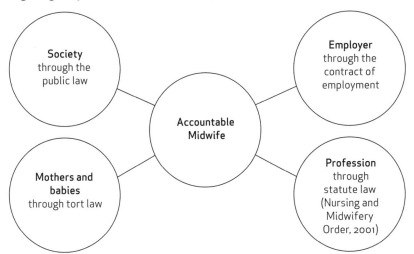

Activity 3.4   *Critical thinking*

A student midwife attacked her former boyfriend's mother with a claw hammer after the relationship broke down. She blamed her for encouraging her son to see another woman. She telephoned the ex-boyfriend's mother and went to see her to talk about her failed relationship. But when the mother left the room and bent to put on her shoes, she attacked her 'like a woman possessed', striking her seven or eight times on the head with the hammer. Despite the woman's screams, the student midwife continued to hit her. She sustained severe injuries and was hospitalised for over three weeks.

The day before the attack, the student had pasted photos of her ex-boyfriend around the estate where he lives with the words 'cheat' and 'liar' on them.

- Using Figure 3.1, list the bodies that may hold the student midwife to account and the possible sanctions they might bestow.

A brief outline answer is given at the end of the chapter.

Accountability to oneself

Often, midwives argue that they are accountable to themselves for their acts and omissions. Such an argument is characteristic of the altruistic nature of the profession. There is no question that a midwife who harms a mother or baby through their acts or omissions will feel remorse and will reflect on their practice to prevent a recurrence. However, this cannot be regarded as a midwife truly holding themselves to account as they cannot apply sanctions and provide any redress to the person who has been wronged.

The authorities mentioned in Figure 3.1 protect the public through the powers conferred on them by the law and can apply sanctions to a midwife who fails to meet the standard imposed by the law.

The spheres of accountability are not mutually exclusive. They can individually or collectively impose sanctions on midwives who fail to meet the required legal standard.

Where misconduct is particularly serious, all four spheres of accountability will come to bear against the midwife.

CASE STUDY: Timesheet fraud

A supervisor of midwives pleaded guilty to falsifying timesheets, costing the NHS more than £63,000 (NHSBSA, 2009). She pleaded guilty to 16 charges of theft and fraud and agreed to a further 28 counts being taken into consideration. She was sentenced to 15 months in prison and ordered to pay £63,812 in compensation. She was dismissed from her job and the NMC will hold her to account on her release from jail.

Accountability to society

As individuals working in the UK, midwives are subject to the same laws as other members of society. If you are suspected of committing a crime during the course of your practice or otherwise, society will hold you to account through the public law.

Many of these laws are derived from Acts of Parliament, such as the Theft Act 1968, the Offences Against the Person Act 1861, the Mental Capacity Act 2005 or the Fraud Act 2006. These Acts are known as public general Acts and it is entirely possible to breach them in the course of your practice. Breaching a provision of a public general Act usually attracts a criminal charge where you have to answer for your actions in a court of law.

Accountability to mothers and babies

As well as being accountable to society in general, midwives are also accountable to the individuals under their care. The tort or civil law system allows redress, usually in the form of compensation, if a woman or her baby has been harmed by a midwife's carelessness.

In the NHS, clinical negligence claims for maternity care amounted to some £226 million in 2009 (NHSLA, 2009).

The legal expression of the ethical principle of non-maleficence is given in the law of negligence. A fundamental principle of healthcare ethics is that midwives should do no harm to the women and babies in their care. Therefore, where harm occurs as the result of a midwife's carelessness, redress in the form of compensation can be sought through the tort or civil law system. Negligence is a civil wrong or tort and is best defined as actionable harm – that is, a person sues for compensation because they have been harmed by the careless act of another person as seen in the case study below.

CASE STUDY: £3 million payout for negligence

In *Wisniewski v Central Manchester HA* [1998], a girl left with a severe disability due to oxygen starvation during her birth received a £3 million compensation payout when the hospital admitted that a delay in delivery caused her brain damage. Had the midwife called a doctor to carry out an assisted delivery just 15 minutes earlier, the girl would have escaped permanent injury.

That delay meant that she suffered acute hypoxia and cerebral palsy. She will need an enormous amount of care and assistance for as long as she lives.

The case study illustrates that careless action, or inaction, by a midwife can result in compensation that runs to several million pounds (see also Chapter 10).

Accountability to the employer

Midwives are accountable to their employer through the contract of employment. The contract sets out the terms and conditions of employment and the standard of work expected of the employee (Rideout, 1983). Many of these terms (e.g. salary, holiday entitlement, hours of work) are written in the contract and are known as 'express contract terms'. In addition, many conditions that regulate the relationship between employer and employee are not expressly written into the contract, but are there by virtue of decided cases or employment-related legislation. These are known as 'implied contract terms' and include a warranty from the employee to the employer that they will carry out their duties with due care and diligence.

An employer is vicariously liable for the actions of its employees. So, if an employee commits a civil wrong in the course of their employment, it is the employer who is liable to pay any compensation. Employers will wish to minimise the likelihood of that liability arising and are entitled under contract law to hold their employees to account through reasonable disciplinary procedures.

For midwives, their employer is the most likely authority to hold them to account. There are two reasons for this. First, a woman with a grievance against a midwife is more likely to complain to the employing Trust than take legal action. Second, employment law allows a lower burden of proof when deciding whether an employee is guilty of misconduct.

In criminal law, the prosecution must prove beyond reasonable doubt that a person is guilty of an offence. In civil law, the person must show on the balance of probability that a tort was committed against them. Employment law only requires that an employer hold an honest and genuine belief that the employee is guilty of misconduct based on the outcome of a reasonable investigation (*British Home Stores Ltd v Burchell* [1980]). This means that, even though a criminal investigation or civil claim may not be successful, action can still be taken by an employer. This is illustrated in the next case study.

CASE STUDY: *Nurse accused of rape*

A registered nurse was accused of raping a pensioner and indecently assaulting another woman while they were patients at a hospital where he worked. However, he was cleared of rape at trial and was never charged with the second assault as police found no DNA evidence at the scene.

Despite being found not guilty, he was dismissed by the employing Trust for gross misconduct. He appealed against the dismissal on the grounds that he was not convicted of an offence, but lost an unfair dismissal claim at an employment tribunal because the Trust held an honest and genuine belief that he was guilty of misconduct. He was also later struck off the register by the NMC for professional misconduct, as they were satisfied on the balance of probability that his conduct was unworthy of a registered nurse (Bourke, 2005, p21).

Midwives who breach their contract by failing to follow reasonable procedures and policies, or who do not work with due care and diligence, can be held to account by their employer even where their actions do not amount to a crime, civil wrong or professional misconduct.

Accountability to the profession

Registered midwives are accountable to the profession through the provisions of the Nurses, Midwives & Health Visitors Act 1997 and the Nursing and Midwifery Order 2001. The NMC was established under these provisions in 2002 and, as the regulatory body for the profession, is concerned with protecting the public.

The key to the NMC's role is the professional register, where the names of those entitled to be called registered midwives are maintained. An active registration is required if a midwife intends to practise. The NMC protects the public by controlling entry on to the register through standards of training and education (NMC, 2009e) and regulating a practitioner's right to remain on the register by imposing professional standards.

'Fitness to practise' is the term used by the NMC to describe a registrant's suitability to be on the register without restrictions. The NMC has the power to hold registered midwives, including independent midwives, to account if it is alleged that their fitness to practise is impaired. Fitness to practise may be impaired by:

- misconduct;
- lack of competence;
- a conviction or caution (including a finding of guilt by a court martial);
- physical or mental ill health;
- a finding by any other health or social care regulator or licensing body that a registrant's fitness to practise is impaired;
- a fraudulent or incorrect entry in the NMC's register.

The standards by which practitioners are judged, and that the NMC considers the public are entitled to expect, are set out in *The Code: Standards of conduct, performance and ethics for nurses and midwives* (NMC, 2008a). Practitioners who appear before the NMC's fitness to practise panels are held to account against those standards. The standards of conduct and competence expected by the NMC are those of the average practitioner, not the highest possible level of practice. This approach is similar to that adopted by the civil law when judging a skilled practitioner under the *Bolam* test to determine whether liability in negligence has arisen (see Chapter 10). The key difference between the law of negligence and professional accountability is that no action in negligence can occur without harm to the patient. A breach of *The Code* can occur, and a midwife be held to account, even without harm to a patient.

The NMC (2004c) admits it would be impossible to compile a definitive list of the type of breaches of *The Code* investigated. However, cases regularly considered include:

- physical, sexual or verbal abuse;
- theft;
- failure to provide adequate care (for registrants who are employers and managers, this can include failing to maintain an acceptable environment of care);
- failure to keep proper records;
- failure to administer medicines safely;
- deliberately concealing unsafe practice;
- committing criminal offences;
- continued lack of competence despite opportunities to improve.

As the NMC is concerned with public safety, the degree of misconduct must reach a level that gives rise to concern for the safety of the public. This often means that a midwife called to account by the NMC for professional misconduct faces several charges that, taken together, give rise to a concern for public safety. The NMC expects the midwife's employer to take appropriate disciplinary action where lesser matters of misconduct, such as arriving late for work, are concerned.

CASE STUDY: Protecting public safety

A midwife was struck off the professional register because of incompetence and misconduct. She failed to meet key objectives during a period of supervised practice with regard to communication, record keeping and lack of care when administering medication.

The Conduct and Competence Committee was told that, while on duty as a midwife on the labour ward, she incorrectly administered intravenous insulin to a woman in the belief that she was administering an epidural top-up and failed to have medication checked by a second midwife (NMC, 2010b).

Midwifery rules and standards

The Nursing and Midwifery Order 2001 requires the NMC to maintain a register of midwives and set out standards of proficiency to be met by those on the register. The NMC sets out rules and standards for midwifery practice and for the statutory supervision of midwives. This means that, as well as having to abide by the requirements of The Code (2008a), midwives can also be held to account where they fail to meet the standards set out in the Midwives Rules and Standards (NMC, 2004b). There are 16 rules and standards set out by the NMC that describe what is reasonably to be expected from a person who practises as a midwife.

- **Rule 1: Citation and commencement**
  This rule sets out that the rules may be cited as the NMC (Midwives) Rules and the commencement date is 1 August 2004.
- **Rule 2: Interpretation**
  This rule describes and offers guidance on the terminology used in the document. For example, there are definitions of childbirth, local supervising authority midwifery officer, practising midwife, supervisor of midwives, etc. As a student midwife, if you are uncertain about the meaning of a professional term, this is where you will find the authoritative definition.
- **Rule 3: Notification of intention to practise**
  A registered midwife must notify the local supervising authority within whose area they intend to practise before they can begin to practise.
- **Rule 4: Notification by local supervising authority**
  The local supervising authorities, who are charged with ensuring that the statutory supervision of midwives is carried out, use the completed intention to practise forms to support and develop midwives in their area, to ensure that practice is up to date.
- **Rule 5: Suspension from practice by a local supervising authority**
  A local supervising authority (the Strategic Health Authorities (SHAs) in England, the Health and Social Services boards in Northern Ireland, the Regional Boards in Scotland and the Health Inspectorate in Wales) may suspend a midwife from practice if there is cause for concern over his or her fitness to practise.

- **Rule 6: Responsibility and sphere of practice**
  A practising midwife is responsible for providing midwifery care in accordance with standards set out by the NMC and must not provide any care or treatment, other than in an emergency, that they have not been trained to give. Where there is an emergency, appropriate qualified health professionals should be called upon for assistance (see Chapter 10).
- **Rule 7: Administration of medicines**
  A practising midwife must only supply and administer medicines they have received appropriate training to administer (see Chapter 13).
- **Rule 8: Clinical trials**
  A practising midwife may only participate in clinical trials where there is a protocol approved by a relevant ethics committee.
- **Rule 9: Records**
  Midwives must keep, as contemporaneously as is reasonable, continuous and detailed records of care given, including administration of medicine, to a woman or baby (see Chapter 8).
- **Rule 10: Inspection of premises and equipment**
  A practising midwife must give a supervisor of midwives, a local supervising authority and the NMC access to records, equipment and place of work (including his or her own residence) in order to monitor standards and methods of practice.
- **Rule 11: Eligibility of appointment as a supervisor of midwives**
  This rule sets out the eligibility for appointment as a supervisor of midwives.
- **Rule 12: The supervision of midwives**
  This rule relates to the supervision of midwives, with guidance about the responsibility of the practising midwife and the role of the local supervising authority.
- **Rule 13: The local supervising authority midwifery officer**
  This rule relates to the appointment of the local supervising authority midwifery officer.
- **Rule 14: Exercise by a supervising authority of its functions**
  Under this rule, the local supervising authority can investigate concerns relating to the supervision of midwives and consult with the NMC as a resource for professional issues.
- **Rule 15: Publication of local supervising authority procedures**
  The local supervising authority shall publish its procedures in dealing with matters relating to midwifery practice, including supervision, grievance, complaints, etc.
- **Rule 16: Annual reports**
  Under this rule each local supervising authority shall submit an annual report to the council to include the number of supervisors in post, how midwifery practice is supervised, complaints, etc. This will enable the NMC to monitor that the local supervising authority is meeting the required standards.

Activity 3.5	Research and group work

Download a copy of the NMC *Midwives Rules and Standards* at **www.nmc-uk.org**. Read each standard and the related guidance. Discuss with colleagues how these relate to your practice as a midwife. You may refer to a relevant chapter in this book. For example, when discussing the importance of a good standard of record keeping (standard 9), you could refer to Chapter 9.

As the answer will be based on your own ideas and experience, there is no outline answer at the end of the chapter.

Statutory supervision of midwives

Supervision of midwives is a statutory responsibility under the Nursing and Midwifery Order 2001 and the NMC *Midwives Rules and Standards* (2004b). It provides a mechanism for supporting and guiding practising midwives in the UK through supervision in order to promote a safe standard of midwifery practice and protect women and babies (NMC, 2008a). All practising midwives, whether hospital, community based or independent of the NHS, are legally required to be supervised.

The statutory requirement that midwives be supervised can be traced to the Midwives Act 1902, which protected the title 'midwife' and set requirements for certification and entry on to the roll of midwives. Supervision under the 1902 Act was undertaken by local councils, with health authorities only taking over the role on creation of the NHS (NHS Act 1946, section 23). Now the role is undertaken by the local supervising authorities (LSAs), who are responsible for the supervision of all midwives within their geographical area. In England the LSAs are Strategic Health Authorities (SHAs); in Scotland and Northern Ireland they are the Health Boards. In Wales the Health Inspectorate fulfils the role. Each authority has an appointed midwifery officer (local supervising authority midwifery officer, or LSAMO) who oversees the supervision of practising midwives. This supervision is undertaken by experienced practising midwives, with at least three years' experience, who have successfully completed an approved NMC education programme to become a supervisor of midwives (SoM). They are accountable to the LSAMO.

The aim of statutory supervision has always been to promote best practice, prevent poor practice and intervene in unacceptable practice. Supervisors of midwives provide advice, guidance and support to individual midwives in relation to practice issues, and ensure that they comply with the *Midwives Rules*.

CASE STUDY: *Midwife stood by as baby's head turned blue*

A midwife who left a newborn baby under water for 15 minutes before calling for help was struck off by the NMC (Knowles, 2009).

The midwife left the mother and baby during advanced labour as the child's head turned blue in a birthing pool. Supervisors had to step in to resuscitate the infant. During another incident the midwife had left a nervous student midwife to untangle a baby's umbilical cord from around its neck and only stepped in to help when the mother hurled abuse at her. The midwife then went into a cupboard to fill in her notes, leaving the student to deal with the birth.

While the supervisor of midwives can step in and respond to incidents of poor practice, and while LSAs have the authority to suspend midwives in their area who fall below the standards required by the *Midwives Rules*, it is the NMC that is charged with investigating the fitness to practise of a midwife.

Investigation of complaints

Everyone has the right to make a complaint to the NMC. The NMC receives complaints from practitioners, other health professions, patients and their families, employers, managers and the public. The police are required to notify the NMC of any registered practitioner convicted of a criminal offence.

Allegations of unfitness to practise are dealt with by three NMC committees.

The Investigating Committee

Once an allegation of unfitness to practise is received by the NMC, it is initially considered by a panel of the Investigating Committee. These private hearings consider the merits of a case by reviewing the available evidence and have the power to recommend what further action needs to be taken.

The Health Committee

A midwife's fitness to practise can be affected by her health as well as her conduct and competence. The Health Committee will determine whether a registered midwife is not fit to practise due to a health concern. In 2008–09 some 22 nurses and midwives (the NMC does not separate the professions in its statistics) were suspended from the professional register on health grounds, mainly due to mental health problems and the misuse of alcohol or drugs (NMC, 2009a).

Conduct and Competence Committee

Panels of the Conduct and Competence Committee consider allegations that have been referred to them by the Investigating or Health Committees. A panel consists of three people with at least one member of the panel having expertise in the same area of practice and being on the same part of the register as the practitioner appearing before it.

Conduct and Competence Committee hearings are held in public, reflecting the NMC's public accountability, although parts of the case may be held in private to protect the anonymity of a victim or disclosure of confidential medical evidence. The panels are advised on points of law and issues of evidence by a legal assessor. The accused is now generally represented by a trade union officer or a lawyer. Where the practitioner chooses not to attend and is not represented, the panel has the power to proceed in their absence.

The Conduct and Competence Committee panel must decide if the case against the accused practitioner is well founded (Nursing and Midwifery Order 2001, art. 29). Since November 2008 cases are determined using the civil standard of proof; that is, on the balance of probabilities.

Sanctions

Where further action needs to be taken, the Nursing and Midwifery Order 2001 allows the NMC to impose a wide range of sanctions to protect the public from midwives whose fitness to practise is impaired.

Sanctions available to the NMC include:

- referring the matter to screeners for mediation;
- deciding that it is not appropriate to take any further action;
- making an order directing the Registrar to strike the person concerned off the register (a 'striking-off order');
- making an order directing the Registrar to suspend the registration of the person concerned for a specified period which shall not exceed one year (a 'suspension order');
- making an order imposing conditions with which the person concerned must comply for a specified period which shall not exceed three years (a 'conditions of practice order');
- cautioning the person concerned for a specified period which shall be not less than one year and not more than five years (a 'caution order').

The NMC's *Fitness to Practise Annual Report* (NMC, 2009f, p12) shows that 210 nurses and midwives were struck off and 126 cautioned to the year ending March 2009. The Case Studies below show a variety of cases involving midwives considered by the NMC in that year.

CASE STUDY: Midwives before the NMC Fitness to Practise Committee

- A midwife gave a woman drugs to induce contractions instead of pain relief when she was already in labour. He should have administered a dose of diamorphine to the mother, but accidentally injected the drug syntometrine. The blunder could have placed both mother and baby at risk as it causes the uterus to contract even more.
- An independent midwife was accused of randomly cutting a woman and her 12lb baby with a pair of scissors. The woman needed extensive surgery after the delivery and her daughter was cut and pulled so forcefully during her birth that the nerves in her neck and arm were severed.
- A midwife was struck off after giving a pregnant woman aromatherapy oils for headache, only for her to drink them by mistake. The woman needed monitoring by the hospital's poisons unit to check for any ill effects, before she later gave birth to a healthy boy.
- A midwife moonlighting as a nurse in a care home was accused of turning off the patient alarms so that she could sleep on night duty.

Source: NMC Fitness to Practise hearings and outcomes (**www.nmc-uk.org/ Hearings/Hearings-and-outcomes**).

Strengthening public confidence in the NMC

The NMC is itself regulated by the Council for Healthcare Regulatory Excellence (CHRE), which oversees the disciplinary decisions of the main bodies of the healthcare professions. It has the power under section 29 of the National Health Service Reform and Health Care Professions Act 2002 to seek a judicial review of a disciplinary decision of a healthcare regulatory body where it considers that decision to be unduly lenient.

The only case yet to be considered by the court in relation to the decisions of the NMC is outlined in the case study below.

CASE STUDY: Lenient punishment

In *Council For The Regulation Of Health Care Professionals v (1) The Nursing And Midwifery Council (2) Steven Truscott* [2004], the Council sought a review of the decision of the NMC to issue a caution to a paediatric nurse who downloaded adult pornographic images while on duty. The Council felt that, although Truscott was dismissed from his job, the decision of the Professional Conduct Committee to give him a caution was unduly lenient.

The Court of Appeal held that the decision of the NMC was lenient but it was not unduly so.

It can be seen that you are accountable to the profession through the provisions of the Nursing and Midwifery Order 2001. This empowers the NMC to maintain a professional register of practitioners and to determine the standards of education and training necessary to enter the register and to establish standards for practice in order to remain on the register. The standards expected of a registered practitioner are set out in *The Code* (NMC, 2008a).

The Code

A revised code of professional conduct was issued by the NMC in March 2008. To make full use of *The Code* it is essential to read its clauses in conjunction with fuller guidance from the NMC in the form of advice sheets. For example, the code requires registered midwives to respect people's confidentiality (see Chapter 9). Fuller information on the extent of this duty is given in the NMC's Confidentiality Advice Sheet, available (like *The Code*) from the NMC's website.

Guidance for students on professional conduct

The NMC (2009c) issues separate guidance on professional conduct for nursing and midwifery students. It outlines what is expected of you while you study to become a registered midwife and prepares you for the obligations you face once qualified. The guidance highlights that, as well as academic success and clinical competence, your behaviour and health during your education are also key components of registration and fitness to practise.

Misconduct, chronic poor health and unhealthy lifestyle choices can lead your university and the NMC to question whether you are fit to practise unsupervised as a registered midwife. This may happen where you have been:

- aggressive, violent or using threatening behaviour;
- cheating or plagiarising work;
- given a criminal conviction or caution;
- dishonest;
- misusing drugs or alcohol;
- having persistent serious health problems;
- persistently inappropriate in your attitude or behaviour;
- guilty of unprofessional behaviour or conduct.

It is essential to follow the guidance throughout your training and to seek guidance and support on any matter that might affect your fitness to practise.

The NMC distributes copies of the guidance to all universities. You can also download copies from the website.

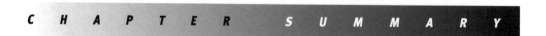

C H A P T E R   S U M M A R Y

- To be accountable is to be answerable for your acts and omissions. You are personally accountable for your practice.
- You are answerable for your acts and omissions regardless of advice or directions from another professional. You do not have control or authority over who holds you to account or what you are accountable for.
- The purpose of accountability is to ensure that the public and patients are not harmed and to provide redress to those who have been harmed. To provide

maximum protection to the public and patients, four areas of law are drawn together and can individually or collectively hold you to account.

- Midwives will not generally be able to argue that they are not accountable because of a lack of experience.
- The regulatory body for the profession is the Nursing and Midwifery Council (NMC), which is concerned with protecting the public.
- Fitness to practise may be impaired by misconduct, lack of competence, a conviction or caution, physical or mental ill health, a finding by any other health or social care regulator or licensing body that a registrant's fitness to practise is impaired, or a fraudulent or incorrect entry in the NMC register.
- The NMC is itself regulated by the Council for Healthcare Regulatory Excellence (CHRE), which oversees the disciplinary decisions of the main regulatory bodies of the healthcare professions.

Activities: brief outline answers

Activity 3.4: Critical thinking (page 39)

The bodies that may hold the student midwife to account, and the possible sanctions they might bestow, are as follows.

- Society through the public law: the student midwife is likely to face a criminal charge of grievous bodily harm. If found guilty, a term of imprisonment is the most likely punishment rather than a fine or community order.
- If she was a registered midwife, she would be accountable to the profession through the Nursing and Midwifery Order 2001. She would be asked to justify her actions by a Conduct and Competence Committee of the NMC. If guilty of professional misconduct, given the seriousness of the allegations, the most likely sanction will be a striking-off order.
- For nursing and midwifery students, the NMC (2009c) has now issued separate guidance on professional conduct. It outlines what is expected of you while you study to become a registered midwife and prepares you for the obligations you face once qualified. The guidance highlights that, as well as academic success and clinical competence, your behaviour during your education is also a key component of registration and fitness to practise. Aggressive and violent behaviour or a criminal conviction or caution can lead the university and the NMC to question whether you are fit to practise unsupervised as a registered midwife.
- If she was a registered midwife employed by an NHS Trust, for example, the employer would hold her to account through the law of contract. An investigation of the incident will be conducted and, if her employer reasonably believes that she is guilty of misconduct, she can be dismissed by her employer for breach of contract.

  As a student midwife, the university and the NMC would question whether she is fit to practise as a registered midwife. She will undoubtedly be held to account by the fitness to practise panel of the university, who may decide to remove her from the course.
- If she has harmed a patient under her care, she could be held to account through the civil law. It will be argued that the Trust caring for the patient breached their duty of care, causing harm, and will be sued for compensation in the civil courts.

Knowledge review

Having completed the chapter, how would you now rate your knowledge of the following topics?

	Good	Adequate	Poor
1. Definitions of the terms 'accountability' and 'responsibility'.			
2. The four spheres of accountability in midwifery practice.			
3. The conduct required to avoid liability in each of these four spheres.			
4. The role of accountability in midwifery.			

Where you're not confident in your knowledge of a topic, what will you do next?

Further reading

NHS Litigation Authority (2009) *Report and Accounts 2008–09*. London: The Stationery Office.
Provides information about the types of claims made against the NHS in England.

Nursing and Midwifery Council (NMC) (2004) *Complaints about Unfitness to Practise: A guide for members of the public*. London: NMC.
Gives you an insight into how the NMC protects the public by encouraging them to report concerns about nurses.

Nursing and Midwifery Council (NMC) (2009) *Fitness to Practice Annual Report*. London: NMC.
It is vital that you understand in practical terms the number and types of cases the NMC deals with in a typical year: a recommended read.

Useful websites

www.nhsbsa.nhs.uk/fraud The NHS Counter Fraud Service.
This organisation is responsible for policy and operational matters relating to the prevention, detection and investigation of fraud in the NHS. Accessing the website enables you to read about individuals who have been held to account because of unlawful conduct.

www.nmc-uk.org Nursing and Midwifery Council.
Essential for all student midwives, here you will find additional guidance, news, consultations for you to contribute to, and dates of fitness to practise hearings (you should make every effort to attend at least once during your training to experience accountability at work).

Chapter 4

Equality and human rights

Chapter aims

After reading this chapter, you will be able to:

- explain what is meant by a 'right';
- describe the purpose of the Human Rights Act 1998 and discuss how it affects the delivery of maternity and child health services;
- outline the measures public organisations must take to comply with their legal obligations;
- illustrate the measures enacted to prohibit discrimination;
- state the role of the Equality and Human Rights Commission.

Introduction

This chapter explores the notion of rights as they apply to midwifery and will focus in particular on human rights. The provisions and key concepts of the Human Rights Act 1998 are introduced and discussed, with the emphasis on how the shift to a rights-based legal system has affected midwifery practice. Leading on from this, the chapter highlights how the state's obligations under the Human Rights Act 1998 have resulted in stronger laws protecting people from discrimination. Disability discrimination and race discrimination are explored in the context of healthcare.

A right is an interest recognised and protected in law. The traditional method of bestowing rights in the legal systems of the UK is to place obligations on others to act or refrain from acting in a particular way. For example, women have a right not to be harmed when in your care. You have an obligation – a legal duty – to be careful when attending women. Where you fail in that duty and cause harm to a woman you will be liable in the law of negligence. In the UK, Parliament is able to create, remove and change the laws and the obligations imposed by them. Following the atrocities of the Second World War, the European Convention on Fundamental Rights and Freedoms was created by the Council of Europe to formalise the relationship between individuals and the government of the country in which they live. The main purpose of the Convention is to limit a state's interference with the rights of the citizens, because some rights are considered so fundamental that they must be respected in every individual's case.

Although the UK was an early signatory to the Convention, enforcing human rights was a difficult and protracted process as Parliament had never incorporated the Convention into domestic law. This was changed by the Human Rights Act 1998, making the main provisions of the Convention enforceable in UK law. This marked a constitutional shift in the legal protection of human rights. There is no doubt that the Human Rights Act 1998 has brought about a culture of rights and responsibilities that, over time, will permeate the whole of our institutions and society.

It is not surprising, then, that the Human Rights Act 1998 affects the way healthcare is provided, given that health is not only a priority on the political platform but also a concern for most people.

Activity 4.1   *Research and group work*

Before reading on, write down what you understand by the term 'human rights'. Then, with two or three others, look at the list below, of the main rights incorporated in the Human Rights Act 1998, listed with their article numbers.

  2: Right to Life
  3: Prohibition of Torture
  4: Prohibition of Slavery and Forced Labour
  5: Right to Liberty and Security
  6: Right to a Fair Trial
  7: No Punishment Without Law
  8: Right to Respect for Private and Family Life
  9: Freedom of Thought, Conscience and Religion
 10: Freedom of Expression
 11: Freedom of Assembly and Association
 12: Right to Marry
 14: Prohibition of Discrimination
 16: Restrictions on Political Activity of Aliens
 17: Prohibition of Abuse of Rights
 18: Limitation on Use of Restrictions on Rights

Select which rights apply to midwifery practice and briefly give some reasons why.

A brief outline answer is given at the end of the chapter.

The Human Rights Act 1998 works by unlocking Convention rights making them enforceable before UK courts and tribunals. It is unlawful for public authorities, including the NHS and the NMC, to act in a way that is incompatible with these rights (Human Rights Act 1998, s6). A good example of how a regulatory body such as the NMC might breach fundamental human rights is illustrated by the following case study, which concerns the NMC's predecessor.

CASE STUDY: Regulatory body breaches human rights

In *Brabazon-Drenning v UK Central Council for Nursing, Midwifery and Health Visiting* [2001], a nurse appealed against a decision to strike her off the Register of Nurses following a disciplinary hearing at which she had not been present. She argued that the hearing ought to have been adjourned because of her unfitness to attend, confirmed by her GP.

The court allowed the appeal as it was a violation of the principles of natural justice and also of the Human Rights Act 1998, schedule 1, part I, article 6 – Right to a Fair Trial – for a committee to continue with a hearing when there was unchallenged medical evidence that the individual was too ill to put her own case.

How the Human Rights Act 1998 works

The laws of the UK continue to apply in the same way. The duties imposed on a midwife when caring for a woman through the laws of negligence, consent and confidentiality continue to be applied. However, where a person, such as an expectant mother, believes that a law or the way a law is enforced breaches a fundamental right of the Convention they can challenge it in court. The courts supervise the decisions of public authorities when human rights are in question (*R (Mahmood) v Secretary of State for the Home Department* [2001]).

The Human Rights Act 1998 requires that all legislation is interpreted and given effect so as to comply with Convention rights regardless of when the Act in question came into force (Human Rights Act 1998, s3). The courts will do their best to apply this principle to avoid the need to change the law.

CASE STUDY: Can an unmarried couple adopt a child?

In *Re P (A Child) (Adoption: Unmarried Couples)* [2008], a couple appealed against a decision rejecting them as prospective adopters because they were unmarried. The court held that the requirement of article 14 of the Adoption (Northern Ireland) Order 1987, that only married or single people could adopt, was discriminatory and contrary to the unmarried couple's right to respect for a private and family life.

The court was free, therefore, to give what it considered to be a principled and rational interpretation of discrimination on grounds of marital status. The court declared that the unmarried couple were entitled to apply to adopt the child and it would be unlawful to reject them as prospective parents only on the grounds that they were not married.

Where the breach of a fundamental human right cannot be remedied by a new interpretation of the existing law, the courts declare that law incompatible with the Human Rights Act 1998 and leave it to Parliament to amend the offending Act (Human Rights Act 1998, s4). This is achieved by Parliament making a remedial order to amend the legislation to bring it into line with the Convention.

Obligations created by the Human Rights Act 1998

Positive obligations

Article 1 of the European Convention on Human Rights requires that steps are taken to secure fundamental rights and freedoms for citizens. This requires a formal relationship between citizens and the state, and creates a positive obligation to ensure that laws and policies are in place to prevent one person violating the human rights of another. Where such law and policies are absent, the victim can take the UK government to court for a breach of their positive obligation.

CASE STUDY: Failure to protect a child from a beating

In *A v UK* [1998], an unruly nine-year-old boy was beaten by his stepfather, who was subsequently charged with assault occasioning actual bodily harm. At trial the stepfather was acquitted after the jury accepted the defence of reasonable chastisement. The boy then took the government to the European Court of Human Rights, alleging a breach of their positive obligation to protect him from inhuman and degrading treatment and punishment under article 3 of the Convention. The Court held that English law failed to protect children as it allowed the defence of reasonable chastisement. The government gave an undertaking to the court that English law would be amended to increase protection.

Negative obligations

A negative obligation requires that a state and its public authorities respect human rights in their day-to-day dealings with individuals. As professionals providing a service on behalf of the state, midwives working for the NHS must exercise their negative obligation by not behaving in a way that would violate the human rights of the women in their care.

Absolute, limited and qualified rights

The European Convention on Human Rights does not contain a list of rights that carry the same weight in law. Rights are categorised by the Convention as absolute, limited or qualified.

Absolute rights

Absolute rights, such as the right to life (article 2), protection from torture, inhuman or degrading treatment or punishment (article 3), and the prohibition on slavery and enforced labour (article 4) may not be deviated from in any circumstances.

CASE STUDY: No-lift policies and human rights

In *R (on the application of A and Others) v East Sussex County Council and Another* [2003], the High Court held that a no-lift policy that completely banned manual handling would be in breach of the right to life (article 2) and a policy that only allowed it where a person's life was in danger would breach the absolute right of freedom from torture, inhuman or degrading treatment or punishment

---

> **CASE STUDY** continued
>
> (article 3). The Court held that, in some circumstances, such as a fire endangering a person's life or where a person might be left for too long in their own excrement or might develop pressure sores if not moved, manual handling might be the only way to protect them from a breach of these fundamental human rights.

Limited rights

Limited rights, such as the right to liberty (article 5), have limited exceptions under explicit and finite circumstances set out in the Convention itself.

For example, if the right to liberty was absolute, the state would not be able to imprison criminals or detain people with mental disorders or diseases who were a danger to public health. Therefore, article 5(1)(a) of the Convention allows for the lawful detention of a person after conviction by a competent court and article 5(1)(e) provides for the lawful detention of persons for the prevention of the spreading of infectious diseases, and of persons of unsound mind.

> **CASE STUDY: A breach of the right to liberty**
>
> In *St George's Healthcare NHS Trust v S* [1998], the Court of Appeal agreed that it was unlawful to detain a woman under the Mental Health Act 1983 simply because she had refused to go to hospital for a caesarean section. The 1983 Act made it clear that its provisions were limited to the treatment of mental disorders and a law that allowed the state to detain a woman for the treatment of an unrelated physical condition would be in breach of the right to liberty under article 5 of the European Convention on Human Rights.

Qualified rights

Qualified rights include the rights to respect for private and family life (article 8), religion and belief (article 9), freedom of expression (article 10), and assembly and association (article 11).

Qualified rights have general exceptions and derogation, that is, relaxation of the legal rule, is allowed where it:

- has its basis in law; and
- is done to secure a permissible aim set out in the relevant article; and
- is necessary in a democratic society to fulfil a pressing social need, pursue a legitimate aim and be proportionate to the aims being pursued.

Proportionality is a principle that requires any interference with a Convention right to be carefully designed to meet the objective in question and to not be arbitrary or unfair.

> **CASE STUDY: Baby removed from mother without court order**
>
> In *R (on the application of G) v Nottingham City Council* [2008], a woman who gave birth in hospital at 2 a.m. was horrified to find that midwives had handed the baby over to social workers who were acting without a court order.
>
> The court found that removing the baby in such circumstances was a breach of the Children Act 1989 and separating a baby from its mother in that way was not in accordance with the law, did not meet a pressing need and was not proportionate. As such, it breached the right to a private and family life of the mother and baby under the Human Rights Act 1998, schedule 1, part 1, article 8.

Human rights and midwifery practice

The right to life (article 2)

The European Court of Human Rights has stated that this right:

> *ranks as one of the most fundamental provisions in the Convention . . . Together with Article 3 . . . it . . . enshrines one of the basic values of the democratic societies making up the Council of Europe.*
>
> (*NHS Trust A v M* [2001])

Article 2 imposes on the state and its authorities a positive obligation to protect the right to life. The state must take appropriate steps to preserve life and this has been recognised in the healthcare context.

The purpose of article 2 is to emphasise the principle of the sanctity of life. The only inroad into the sanctity of human life it allows has been the withholding of life-sustaining treatment. In the context of midwifery practice, a midwife might be confronted with a situation where a pregnant woman presents at 22 weeks' gestation with a spontaneous rupture of membranes. There are two possible outcomes here: first, the pregnant woman may be counselled about the consequences of giving birth to a very premature baby, such as a low rate of survival and a 50 per cent risk of disability. It would be entirely up to the pregnant woman whether she wishes to terminate the pregnancy as permitted under the Abortion Act 1967. Second, the pregnant woman may have given birth prematurely where the infant is born alive. The infant has a right to life under article 2 as well as rights under the Children Act 1989. Both measures support the maintenance of life in children unless it would not be in the interests of the child to do so.

The remit of article 2 is extremely narrow. It is only engaged when there is intentional or careless human intervention to end life. In cases of withdrawal of treatment for neonates, it would depend on medical advice as to whether this is in the best interests of the child.

> **CASE STUDY: Withdrawing treatment**
>
> In *K (A Child) (Withdrawal of Treatment)* [2006], a Trust sought a declaration allowing doctors to remove a feeding tube and palliative care from a baby to allow her to die peacefully within a short period of time. She had been born prematurely with an inherited condition causing chronic muscle weakness. She experienced

severe feeding difficulties. She was in the worst category of the condition and the issue was not whether she would survive but how soon she was likely to die.

The court gave the declaration as there was no realistic hope that she would have the simple pleasure of being alive or of having anything other than a life dominated by regular pain, distress and discomfort. She had no prospect of relief from her pitiful existence before an end that was regarded as virtually certain by the age of one year, and was likely to be appreciably less. If the feeding line remained in place, she would continue to suffer pain and distress from the invasive treatment that she already experienced, while if she were to have the necessary operation to replace the line, she would require mechanical ventilation, which was also invasive and painful. There would be no improvement in her condition or expectation of life. It would therefore be not only a mercy, but in her best interests, to cease to provide feeding so she could die in peace in a comparatively short space of time in the close care of the parents who loved her.

Prohibition of torture, inhuman or degrading treatment or punishment (article 3)

Although an absolute right, article 3 contains three different thresholds, namely torture, inhuman treatment and degrading treatment. For article 3 to be engaged, one of the three thresholds must be breached.

Torture consists of deliberate inhuman treatment, causing very serious and cruel suffering. The threshold for torture was reduced in *Selmouni v France* [1998], when the European Court of Human Rights held for the first time that a sustained beating amounted to torture, not inhuman treatment. The effect of lowering the threshold for torture is to lower the threshold for inhuman and degrading treatment: whereas few people would claim to have been tortured, many more could argue that their treatment was inhuman or degrading in nature.

Indeed, in *Tanko v Finland* [1994], the European Commission on Human Rights refused to exclude the possibility that a lack of proper medical care in a case where someone is suffering from a serious illness could amount to treatment contrary to article 3.

Inhuman treatment or punishment

Inhuman treatment or punishment is less severe than torture. It includes less serious physical assaults, inhuman detention conditions and a lack of proper medical care.

In *D v UK* [1997], the European Court of Human Rights held that to deport a man in the advanced stages of AIDS would be a breach of article 3. Withdrawal of the care, support and treatment he was currently receiving in the UK would have serious consequences and would expose him to a real risk that he would die in distressing circumstances, which would amount to inhuman treatment contrary to Article 3.

Degrading treatment or punishment

Treatment is degrading if it is ill-treatment that is also grossly humiliating. Treatment is capable of being degrading within the meaning of article 3, whether or not it arouses feelings of fear, anguish or inferiority in the victim. It is enough for it to be judged by the standard of right-thinking bystanders as humiliating or debasing the victim, showing a lack of respect for, or diminishing, their human dignity (*R (Burke) v GMC and Others* [2004]).

If a midwife witnessed the degrading treatment of a woman, that would engage the woman's rights under article 3 even if she was too ill or incapable to be aware of the degrading treatment herself.

The healthcare exception

A key exception to the principle of inhuman or degrading treatment applies to the provision of healthcare. In *Herczegfalvy v Austria* (1993), the European Court of Human Rights recognised that it is for medical authorities to decide on the therapeutic methods to be used, if necessary by force, to preserve the physical and mental health of people.

A measure that is a therapeutic necessity cannot be regarded as inhuman or degrading. However, the Court must be satisfied that the medical necessity of the treatment is convincingly shown to exist. According to the Court of Appeal in *R (on the application of N) v M* [2002], this means that:

- the decision to proceed with treatment had to be in accordance with a respected body of professional opinion as set out in *Bolam v Friern HMC* [1957]; and
- be in the best interests of the person.

Both heads of the definition have to be complied with in order to satisfy the burden of proof that the care or treatment is medically necessary.

Therefore, inhuman or degrading treatment must attain a minimum level of severity if it is to fall within the scope of article 3. This level depends on all the circumstances of the case, and concerns fundamental issues of respect, dignity and humanity. Article 3 can apply to healthcare.

Although article 3 has a broader remit than article 2, it still nevertheless requires a high threshold to be crossed before its provisions are engaged. Only where people are subject to the severest forms of unnecessary distress will their rights under article 3 be engaged.

Respect for private and family life, home and correspondence (article 8)

Article 8 concerns the everyday right of individuals to respect for their private and family life, home and correspondence. However, as a qualified right, article 8 allows scope for intrusion into this right on a variety of grounds, including the protection of health. To be justified, any intrusion must be in accordance with the law and be proportionate to the aim being achieved.

The Convention interprets the concept of private life very broadly. In *Pretty v UK* [2002], the European Court of Human Rights held that:

> the concept of 'private life' is a broad term not susceptible to exhaustive definition. It covers the physical and psychological integrity of a person. It can sometimes embrace aspects of an individual's physical and social identity . . . Article 8 also protects a right to personal development, and the right to establish and develop relationships with other human beings and the outside world.

The Court considers that the notion of personal autonomy is an important principle underlying the interpretation of its guarantees. The very essence of the Convention is respect for human dignity and human freedom.

(*Pretty v UK* [2002] 35 EHRR 1 at [61])

As a qualified right, the threshold for engagement is relatively low. Any interference with a person or the way they live their lives needs to be justified and proportionate. The personal autonomy protected by article 8 means that it is for a competent woman, not the midwife or doctor, to decide what treatment they should be given in order to meet their need for dignity and avoid what people would find distressing. A competent woman's article 8 rights to physical and psychological integrity, to autonomy and dignity will therefore prevail over any rights or obligations located in articles 2 and 3. Any positive obligations of the state under articles 2 or 3 necessarily cease at the point at which they would otherwise come into conflict with, or intrude into, the competent person's rights of autonomy and self-determination under article 8 (*R (Burke) v GMC and Others* [2004]).

In order to show that their practice is in accordance with the law, midwives would need to demonstrate that they had followed the specific legal requirements for the care they have undertaken. For example, midwives would need to demonstrate that women had exercised their right to self-determination by obtaining an effective consent before treatment, and that they had carried out that treatment in a manner that reflected the extent of their duty of care towards the woman.

CASE STUDY: IVF and article 8

In *Rose v Secretary of State for Health and Human Fertilisation and Embryology Authority* [2002], it was found that a child whose existence results from artificial insemination using donor sperm is able to rely on their article 8 right to establish their personal paternal identity, which is an important part of their genetic make-up. The sperm donor has no right to respect for family life, but the resultant child does.

Equality and diversity

To promote equality of rights and prevent discrimination, Parliament has enacted a range of statutes to supplement the Human Rights Act 1998. In particular, the law prohibits discrimination on grounds of disability, gender, race, sexual orientation, religion or belief and age. In addition to the legislative measures taken to combat discrimination, there is a duty on the health service as a public body to promote equality in the provision of services. It is essential that midwives are aware of the legal and policy issues that prohibit discrimination.

Sex Discrimination Act 1975

This legislative measure prohibited discrimination on grounds of gender. A claim is made out where the complainant can show that she has been treated less favourably than a man, or applies to a condition or requirement that only a very small proportion of women could comply with. The twin concept of direct or indirect discrimination was embedded in the measure as a means of ensuring that employers did not use strategies to continue discriminating while ostensibly complying with the law. The legislation covers sexual harassment and also applies to men. A number of amendments have been made in order to protect, for example, people of transgender. The Gender Recognition Act 2004 recognises transgender, while the Sex Discrimination (amendment legislation) Regulations 2008 give added protection to transgender people in the areas of provision of goods, services, facilities and premises.

CASE STUDY: Transgender person applies for police post

An employment tribunal held that West Yorkshire Police's refusal of an application for the post of constable by a transgender person amounted to sex discrimination contrary to the Sex Discrimination Act 1975 (*A v West Yorkshire Police* (1999)). The complainant, a male to female transsexual, applied for the post of constable and, as part of the application process, she had to disclose that she was a transsexual. Following the disclosure, she was informed that she could not be employed as part of the job would require her to search females when legally she was a male. The tribunal heard evidence from both parties, but decided that, as a transsexual, she would be able to carry out her duties and that searching was only a small part of those.

Disability Discrimination Act 1995

Some 20 per cent of people of working age are considered by the government to be disabled, as they have a long-term health condition that has an impact on their everyday lives. Such people now have rights under the Disability Discrimination Act (DDA) 1995, enacted to address the discrimination that many disabled people face. Midwives have a significant role in the continuing care and support of disabled women who are pregnant. It is essential that midwives are aware of how the law defines a disability and what constitutes discrimination under the 1995 Act. This will enable them to identify women who are disabled and who will benefit from the provisions of the DDA 1995, and to recognise an action that would be considered discriminatory and would be unlawful.

The purpose of the Disability Discrimination Act 1995

The DDA 1995 makes it unlawful to discriminate against disabled people in such areas as employment, education and access to goods, facilities and services, including health services. Different parts of this legislation came into effect at different times and the original 1995 Act has since been subject to a number of amendments. In April 2005, a new DDA amended existing provisions by bringing a wider range of conditions under the definition. It also extended the duty not to discriminate against disabled people to educational establishments, private clubs and public transport.

Definition of 'disabled'

The DDA 1995, section 1, defines a person as disabled if they have a physical or mental impairment which has a substantial and long-term adverse effect on their ability to carry out normal day-to-day activities.

There are four key elements to the statutory definition.

- It must be due to a physical or mental impairment.
- The impairment must have substantial adverse effects.

- The adverse effects must be long term.
- These adverse effects must affect a person's ability to carry out normal day-to-day activities.

Physical or mental impairment

The term 'physical or mental impairment' is given its ordinary rather than any particular legal meaning. It can be construed by reference to what an ordinary person would regard as a physical or mental impairment. Mental impairment includes learning disabilities and mental illness. A requirement that a mental illness could only be considered if it was clinically well recognised was removed by the DDA 2005, as arguments over diagnosis frequently resulted in a person being excluded from the protection offered by the Act.

The broadening of the definition of physical and mental impairment enables many additional forms of chronic health problems to fall within the provisions of the DDA. A disability can be due to a wide range of impairments including:

- sensory impairments, such as those affecting sight or hearing;
- impairments with fluctuating or recurring effects, such as rheumatoid arthritis, myalgic encephalitis and chronic fatigue syndrome (CFS);
- progressive conditions such as motor neurone disease, muscular dystrophy and dementia;
- cardiovascular diseases including thrombosis, stroke and heart disease;
- developmental impairments such as autistic spectrum disorders, dyslexia and dyspraxia;
- mental impairments including mental illnesses such as depression, schizophrenia, eating disorders and some self-harming behaviours.

It is not always possible to determine whether a condition is a physical or a mental impairment. There may be adverse effects that are both physical and mental in nature, or the effects of a physical nature may stem from an underlying mental impairment, and vice versa. Some conditions such as alcoholism and a tendency to set fires are excluded from the Act.

It is not necessary to consider how impairment was caused. For example, liver disease as a result of alcohol dependency would be impairment within the meaning of the Act, even though alcoholism itself is excluded.

Particular cases or conditions

Progressive conditions

The DDA covers progressive conditions where impairments are likely to become substantial. Where a person has cancer, HIV infection or multiple sclerosis the provisions of the Act apply from the point of diagnosis. A requirement that there had to be a noticeable effect on the person's normal day-to-day activities was removed for these conditions by the DDA 2005. Similarly, a person who is certified as blind or partially sighted by a consultant ophthalmologist, or registered as such with a local authority, is deemed to meet the definition of disability. For all other progressive conditions the person will be treated as disabled from the moment any impairment resulting from the condition first has some effect on their ability to carry out normal day-to-day activities. The effect need not be continuous or substantial. All that needs to be shown is that there is some effect on the person's ability to carry out normal day-to-day activities (DDA 1995, schedule 1, para. 8).

Past disability

The definition of 'disability' and 'disabled' includes those people who were disabled in the past but have now recovered. For example, a person who some years ago suffered a reactive depression following the loss of a loved one, but who has now recovered, is still entitled to protection from discrimination under the DDA 1995, schedule 2.

Definition of 'substantial'

The requirement that an adverse effect on normal day-to-day activities should be substantial reflects the view that a disability goes beyond the normal differences in ability that may exist among people. A substantial effect is one that is more than minor or trivial.

A number of factors need to be taken into account when considering whether or not an impairment is substantial:

- the time taken by a person with an impairment to carry out normal day-to-day activities compared with that taken by a person who did not have the impairment;
- the cumulative effects of an impairment;
- the effect on a person's behaviour;
- the effect of the environment on the impairment;
- any treatment or corrective measures being taken;
- any disfigurement associated with the impairment.

Definition of 'long term'

The definition of disability requires the effect of the impairment to be long term. According to the DDA 1995, schedule 1, para. 2, a long-term effect is one:

- that has lasted at least 12 months; or
- where the total period for which it lasts, from the time of the first onset, is likely to be at least 12 months; or
- that is likely to last for the rest of the life of the person affected.

If an impairment has had a substantial adverse effect on a person's ability to carry out normal day-to-day activities but that effect ceases, it is treated as continuing if it is likely to recur. That is, it is more likely than not that the effect will recur (for example, as in conditions such as rheumatoid arthritis, mental illness and epilepsy).

Ability to carry out normal day-to-day activities

According to the DDA 1995, schedule 1, para. 4, only an impairment that affects a person in one or more of the following ways will be considered as affecting the ability of a person to carry out normal day-to-day activities:

- mobility;
- manual dexterity;
- physical coordination;
- continence;
- ability to lift, carry or otherwise move everyday objects;
- speech, hearing or eyesight;
- memory or ability to concentrate, learn or understand;
- perception of the risk of physical danger.

Day-to-day activities are things people do on a regular or daily basis, such as shopping, reading and writing, talking, watching television, getting washed and dressed, preparing and eating food, housework, walking, travelling and taking part in social activities. They do not include work activities, as work varies from person to person so cannot be regarded as a normal activity. However, many types of work still involve normal activities such as sitting down, standing up, walking, running, talking, writing, making a cup of tea and using everyday objects.

For the purposes of the 1995 Act, fluctuating impairments should be considered in terms of their substantial and long-term effects on the ability to perform daily tasks both at work and away from work.

Discrimination

The purpose of the DDA 1995 is to prohibit discrimination against people with disabilities.

Activity 4.2	Critical thinking and groupwork

- In a group, discuss your understanding of the word discrimination.
- Then discuss how a service provider, such as an NHS hospital, might discriminate against a woman with a disability.

As this activity involves your own experience, there is no outline answer at the end of the chapter.

The word 'discrimination' comes from the Latin *discriminare*, meaning to distinguish between. Discrimination is now taken to be more than distinction; it is an action based on prejudice resulting in unfair treatment of people.

Under the DDA 1995 it is unlawful to discriminate against a disabled person. Discrimination will arise when, for a reason that relates to a disabled person's disability, they are treated less favourably than others to whom that reason does not apply and it cannot be shown that this treatment was justified (DDA 1995, ss5 and 20).

Duties as a service provider

As a service provider, according to the DDA 1995, section 20, it is unlawful for the health service to discriminate against a disabled person in three key ways:

- **refusing service** – in refusing to provide or deliberately not providing any service that is provided to the general public;
- **standard of service** – in the standard of service provided or the manner in which it is provided;
- **terms of service** – in the terms on which a service is provided.

Refusing service

Refusing to serve or not provide a service to a disabled person for any reason related to their disability is discriminatory.

> ### CASE STUDY: Personal assistants refuse access
>
> A disabled woman in labour was denied the right to have her personal assistants at the bedside when giving birth on the grounds that 'visitors' were not allowed access outside visiting hours (Crow, 2003). The assistants were trained to meet her complex social care and personal needs. This refusal amounted to discrimination.

Standard and terms of service

It is unlawful to offer a disabled person a different level of service compared to other people. It is also unlawful to adopt a worse manner or use spurious reasons when caring for disabled people.

Provision of a service to a disabled person on terms that are worse than the terms offered to other people is also unlawful. To charge customers more because they are disabled is unlawful.

Scenario

A wheelchair user books a place at a campsite to pitch her converted caravan, which she is holidaying in with her recently born twins. When she arrives she explains that she needs a wide pitch to allow for wheelchair and pram access. The site manager charges her double rent for the extra room. The court holds that this was discrimination on the grounds of disability and fines the campsite management.

Reasonable adjustments

Making reasonable adjustments to services, premises, employment conditions or courses of education is key to the duty against discrimination under the DDA 1995. Steps must be taken to ameliorate the person's disability so that they are treated with equality.

Each situation must be viewed on a case-by-case basis according to the requirements of the 1995 Act. The House of Lords holds that the DDA 1995 is fundamentally different from the Sex Discrimination Act 1975 and the Race Relations Act 1976. The latter two Acts require people to be treated the same regardless of race or gender. The DDA 1995 does not regard the differences between the disabled and others as irrelevant. It requires reasonable adjustments to be made to cater for the specific needs of the disabled. It does not only permit the favourable treatment of disabled people, it demands it to the extent required to meet the duty to make reasonable adjustments.

There is no longer any justification for failing to make reasonable adjustments under the DDA 1995. Dismissing a person with a disability without attempting to make reasonable adjustments is direct discrimination and can never be justified (DDA 1995, s3A(5)). For example, in *Tudor v Spen Corner Veterinary Centre* (2006), an employment tribunal found that an employer had directly discriminated against an employee, an animal nursing assistant, when they immediately dismissed her after she lost sight in both eyes. The employer had made generalised and stereotypical assumptions about visually impaired people and did not look at the circumstances of the particular case or consider what reasonable adjustments could be made to help the visually impaired person in her role.

Justifying less favourable treatment

There are instances where less favourable treatment of a disabled person could be justified, but less favourable treatment cannot be justified until the duty to provide reasonable adjustments has been complied with.

To justify less favourable treatment of a disabled person it must be shown that reasonable adjustments cannot be made on the grounds of:

- health and safety;
- inability to give an informed consent;
- inability to enter into an enforceable agreement;
- inability to provide a service to others by serving the disabled person;
- necessity to provide service on different terms in order to serve the disabled person and others;
- greater expense.

CASE STUDY: No paid time off to look after baby

In *Murphy v Slough* [2004], a teacher suffered from a congenital heart disorder, which meant that if she became pregnant and miscarried there was a 50 per cent chance of her dying, so she entered into a surrogacy arrangement in order to have a child. After the child was born she sought paid postnatal leave. The school governors decided that she was only entitled to unpaid leave since the school was in a precarious financial position. The teacher argued that she was being treated less favourably for a reason that related to her disability.

The tribunal found that the teacher had been treated less favourably than other women who gave birth in the normal way to their own children. The reason for the less favourable treatment was due to her disability. However, the school's decision not to grant paid leave was justified on the grounds of the school's difficult financial position.

Discrimination by association

In *Coleman v Attridge Law* [2008], the European Court of Justice ruled that the prohibition of direct discrimination against and harassment of disabled people was intended to protect not only persons who were themselves disabled but also those who cared for disabled people. This means that a woman who loses her job because she has to take considerable time off work to attend hospital with her disabled baby would be subject to disability discrimination by association.

General duty of public bodies

Disability equality duty

There is a legal duty on all public sector organisations to promote equality of opportunity for disabled people. This disability equality duty applies to the NHS and covers the full range of what public sector organisations do, including policy making and services that are delivered to the public. It requires public authorities, when carrying out their functions, to have due regard to the following needs.

- **To promote equality of opportunity between disabled people and other people.** For example, midwives may find that people with learning disabilities are generally poor attendees at clinics. Those responsible for delivering the clinic programme will have to ensure that the service is designed to offer the same opportunities to disabled people as to others. This could be done by working together to look at how the disability equality duty can be met. A key part of this work would involve drawing on advice from people with learning disabilities on how clinics could be made more accessible. An impact assessment would also help to identify what aspects of the clinics may disadvantage people with disabilities.

- **To eliminate discrimination that is unlawful under the DDA 1995.** This reinforces the reasonable adjustment duties of the DDA 1995. It complements the existing anticipatory duty to make reasonable adjustments, requiring adjustments to be made in advance of disabled people attempting to use the service.
- **To eliminate disability-related harassment.** This will require health organisations to have an anti-harassment policy and ensure that staff receive training in disability equality and managing disabled people, including those in distress.
- **To promote positive attitudes towards disabled people.**
- **To encourage participation by disabled people in public life.**
- **To take steps to take account of disabled persons' disabilities, even where that involves treating disabled persons more favourably than other persons.** For example, if a hospital trust allows cancer patients who travel regularly to hospital for treatment to be exempt from hospital car parking charges, they would be treating cancer patients more favourably than non-disabled people, but this could be justified on the grounds of ensuring such frequent clinic attendees have fair access to services.

Public authorities must have published a Disability Equality Scheme that must include:

- a statement of how disabled people have been involved in developing the scheme;
- an action plan that includes practical ways in which improvements will be made;
- the arrangements in place for gathering information about how the public sector organisation has performed in meeting its targets on disability equality.

Race equality duty

Discrimination on grounds of race, ethnicity, colour and national origin can have devastating consequences for the individual concerned and can lead to exclusion from full participation in society. For example, there is higher unemployment among working-age Bangladeshi and Pakistani women who are four times more likely to be unemployed than white British women. This exclusion can in turn lead to poverty and poor health (Nazroo, 2001).

Staff also have the right not to be discriminated against on the grounds of race. A midwife who complained of persistent racial discrimination received £47,000 compensation when a tribunal found that her employing Trust did not take her concerns seriously and failed to carry out an investigation (Dimond, 2006).

> **CASE STUDY: Black nurse told not to treat white baby**
>
> A nurse who was moved to different wards after a mother objected to her child being treated by a black woman won her claim of racial discrimination and received £20,000 in compensation (Payne, 2004). The nurse had been subjected to racist abuse from the mother for seven years. Instead of tackling the source, her employers moved her to other wards at the hospital to prevent her coming into contact with the mother, whose child required regular treatment for cystic fibrosis.

Discrimination on the grounds of race was outlawed by the Race Relations Act 1976, which emphasised the commitment of the UK to eliminate discrimination and promote equal opportunity. The Act empowered individuals to seek justice in cases of perceived or actual discrimination on the grounds of race.

Treating someone less favourably because of race is unlawful. Racial grounds include colour, race, nationality or ethnic or national origins. The Act requires the complainant to point out the discriminatory act but does not require the individual to be named. Segregation on racial grounds is regarded as treating people less favourably. For example, if a midwife insisted that all Asian women were accommodated in a separate bay from other women, she would be acting unlawfully and in a directly discriminatory manner.

The Race Relations Act 1976 also forbids indirect discrimination where a condition or requirement disproportionately affects people from an ethnic or racial background. The Act also prohibits victimisation of a complainant by treating them less favourably because they have brought proceedings under the Act for race discrimination.

Institutional racism

The murder of Stephen Lawrence highlighted the institutional aspect of discrimination. An inquiry into the way the police handled the investigation into the murder concluded that the failures of the police were due to institutional racism. It defined institutional racism as:

> *The collective failure of an organisation to provide an appropriate and professional service to people because of their colour, culture or ethnic origin which can be seen or detected in processes, attitudes and behaviour which amount to discrimination through unwitting prejudice, ignorance, thoughtlessness and racist stereotyping which disadvantages minority ethnic people.*
>
> (Macpherson, 1999)

The inquiry resulted in the Race Relations Amendment Act 2000, which imposed a positive obligation on public bodies, including the NHS, to promote race equality in all areas of their work by placing due regard on the need to:

- eliminate unlawful discrimination;
- promote equality of opportunity and good relations between persons of different racial groups.

The duty is mandatory and must be applied to all functions that are relevant to race equality.

All health services are required to demonstrate how they will comply with their obligations under the Race Relations Amendment Act 2000 through a Race Equality

Scheme. This includes the requirement to assess the impact of a health service's policies on race equality and to demonstrate steps taken to prohibit racial discrimination and promote equal opportunities.

Accessing healthcare

People from ethnic minority communities tend not to make full use of health services compared to the population as whole. According to Nazroo (2001), the reasons include:

- some people not having English as their first language and finding it difficult to know what services are available, or to communicate with health professionals where they do use services;
- cultural difficulties; for example, many Asian women do not accept a consultation with a male doctor and are reluctant to take up cervical and breast screening services;
- cultural beliefs about, and tendency to use, traditional medicines and therapies;
- cultural pressures to hide mental illness and some other illnesses;
- the greater likelihood of people from ethnic minority groups being unemployed or on low income and, therefore, as a group being more susceptible to the health disadvantages related to poverty, including poorer access to healthcare.

Equality Act 2010

The government has consolidated the law on discrimination so that there is a single, modern, piece of legislation that is easy to understand and provides clear guidance about people's rights and responsibilities. The Equality Act comes into force in October 2010. It is important that midwives are aware of the key provisions of the Act in order to inform their practice and ensure that they do not breach any aspect of the revised discrimination legislation.

The three existing public sector equality duties of race, disability and gender have now been brought together and extended to cover religion or belief, sexual orientation and age. The 2010 Act has broad application and applies to employment relationships, to the provision of goods and services, and to public bodies, such as the health service, in exercising their functions.

Key provisions

In order to simplify and strengthen discrimination law, the Equality Act 2010 brings together the existing anti-discrimination provisions contained in current legislation. For example, the protected characteristics of age, disability, gender reassignment, marriage and civil partnership, pregnancy and maternity, race, religion or belief, sex and sexual orientation, which are currently covered by different laws, have been brought under one Act of Parliament. In addition, it extends discrimination law to novel areas and includes new provisions relating to the supply of goods and services and to the way public bodies exercise their functions.

> **Concept summary: Key provisions of the Equality Bill 2010**
>
> - Includes a duty on public bodies to consider reducing social and economic inequalities when taking strategic decisions.

Concept summary continued

- Extends definitions of discrimination to include discrimination by association or false perception.
- Allows employers to take positive actions in terms of under represented groups.
- Extends the circumstances in which a person is protected against discrimination because of a protected characteristic.
- Allows people to make a claim if they are directly discriminated against because of a combination of two protected characteristics.
- Makes it unlawful to discriminate against adults because of their age when providing goods, facilities and services.
- Includes new measures to address pay inequality in the workplace.
- Covers discrimination relating to the use of pre-employment health questionnaires.
- Includes new powers of employment tribunals to make recommendations.

Socioeconomic inequalities

Public bodies must now consider how their decisions might help to reduce socio-economic disadvantage when making strategic decisions. The duty will require public bodies to take into account discrepancies, such as health inequalities and the postcode lottery, during everyday work and while planning and developing new healthcare provision.

An NHS body, such as a Primary Care Trust (PCT) or Local Health Board, may decide that people from a particular socioeconomic background might not be able to access a service provided by midwives during working hours. They would act to reduce this inequality of access by providing a service that meets the needs of those who are disadvantaged. A person cannot sue for damages where there is a breach of this statutory duty, but they can bring judicial review proceedings against the NHS where they believe that socioeconomic disadvantage has not been considered in its strategic decision making.

Discrimination

The Equality Act 2010 replaces the definitions of direct discrimination in current legislation by removing the requirement for the victim to have a protected characteristic such as age, gender or disability.

A person can be directly discriminated against even if they do not have one of the protected characteristics. For example, where a midwife is disciplined for refusing to carry out instructions to exclude teenage mothers from a therapeutic group, this would be direct age discrimination against the midwife unless the instruction can be justified.

The Act also extends discrimination to people who are wrongly perceived to possess any of the protected characteristics. For example, if a midwifery manager rejects an application from a white person whom she wrongly thinks is black (because of her name, for example), this would still be direct race discrimination based on the manager's mistaken perception.

There are also new provisions to correct the erosion of protection intended for disabled people by the DDA 1995, following a House of Lords opinion in the case of *Mayor and Burgesses of the London Borough of Lewisham v Malcolm* [2008]. In that case the claim of a schizophrenic patient that he was treated less favourably because of his disability was overruled by the House of Lords because they found that an able person would have been treated in the same way.

The Equality Act 2010 now provides that discrimination will occur where a person is treated less favourably and it is known or ought reasonably to have been known that the person had a disability. For example, if a person with a known learning disability is asked to leave a midwifery clinic waiting room because they are noisy, that would be discrimination. However, if a person is asked to leave a clinic because they are noisy and it was not at that time known they had a disability, that would not be discrimination.

Positive action

The Equality Act 2010 allows employers to take under-representation in the workforce, such as gender or race, into account when selecting for appointment or promotion between two equally qualified candidates. Guidance on how to apply positive action will be offered by the Equality and Human Rights Commission.

An employer would be entitled to favour the candidate from the under-represented or disadvantaged group, such as those from an ethnic minority group. Employers will also have a defence of 'occupational requirement', where they can show that a particular characteristic is a requirement of the job. For example, an employer can seek applications for a job in a women's refuge from female midwives only.

The European Court of Justice has long held that, although the UK was wrong to grant an exemption from the Sex Discrimination Act 1975 to employment in private houses, an exemption that midwifery should be predominantly a female occupation was not unlawful, as respect for private life is a fundamental principle of the Community, which may justify exemption from a directive laying down rules for enforcing equality of treatment (*Commission of the European Communities v UK (C165/82) [1984]*).

Combined discrimination: dual characteristics

The Equality Act 2010 now includes direct discrimination because of the combination of two protected characteristics, also known as dual discrimination. Therefore, a person might be discriminated against based on a combination of two characteristics such as age and race. The person must show that the alleged discrimination was because of the combination of two characteristics. A comparison has to be made to the treatment of a person who does not share either of the characteristics in the combination. For example, a midwife who treats young black women less favourably than white women or older black women would be guilty of dual discrimination.

Age discrimination in the provision of goods and services

The Equality Act 2010 makes it unlawful to discriminate against adults aged over 18 because of their age when providing goods, facilities and services and carrying out public functions. A midwife will not be able to refuse to provide a service based on age without lawful or medical justification. The provision of products or services for people of different ages will not be affected where this is justified, such as providing breast screening to women over 50. Age discrimination includes people in an age group who are being treated less favourably. For example, if a midwifery service refuses to provide care to women over 40 who are pregnant, that would be age discrimination.

The extension of age discrimination to goods and services has been hailed by critics of the health services as a vital tool to combat ageism in the NHS.

In their review of age equality in health and social care, Carruthers and Ormondroyd (2009) found that:

- age discrimination remains an issue for health and social care services;
- most examples of age discrimination are indirect, but these have just as detrimental an impact;
- the extension of age discrimination to the provision of health and social care should come into force at the same time as for other sectors; currently this will be 2012;
- negative attitudes and narrow assumptions about age, particularly about older people, are an important cause of age discrimination;
- discriminatory behaviour often contributes to poor-quality care: tackling age discrimination is necessary for achieving high-quality care;
- the distribution of resources within the health and social care system will need to conform to the new legislative requirements, and in some situations will require a redistribution of resources so that needs are met more fairly.

Such is the extent of age discrimination in the health service that it was feared that the government would either have to delay the application of this provision to the health service for several years in order to give the NHS time to change its systems and services, or exclude the NHS altogether (Williams, 2009).

Pre-employment medical questions

A new clause was included in the Equality Act 2010 following pressure from disability rights groups, the RCN and the medical royal colleges. The clause will make it unlawful to ask job applicants disability and health questions before a job offer, except in prescribed circumstances. Pre-employment medical questions will still be permitted, such as where an employer might have to take reasonable measures in order to ensure that an applicant who is deaf is not disadvantaged at interview. Employers will need to be careful about what questions are asked at any stage of the recruitment process and be clear about the purpose for asking such questions.

Employment tribunals

Many employees have recourse to an employment tribunal in cases of unfair dismissal due to unfair employment practices such as discrimination. At present, tribunals make recommendations relating to the individual claimants, but if they have left their job the recommendations have no benefit for the other employees. The Equality Act 2010 will allow employment tribunals to make wider recommendations in discrimination cases that will benefit the wider workforce and help to prevent similar types of discrimination occurring in the future.

Equality and Human Rights Commission

The Equality and Human Rights Commission (EHRC, 2007) has extensive legal powers and a team of lawyers who are specialists in equality law. It is equipped to take legal action on behalf of individuals, especially where these are test cases that will test the boundaries of the law and are likely to have a wide impact. Where there are chances to create legal precedents or to clarify and improve the law, the Commission will seek to do so. Unless there is an equality dimension, the Commission is unable to assist individuals in human rights cases. However, it is able to hold formal inquiries or to take judicial review proceedings to prevent breaches of the Human Rights Act 1998, and it can also join in with cases taken by others to promote human rights.

C H A P T E R   S U M M A R Y

- The Human Rights Act 1998 incorporates the main provisions of the European Convention on Human Rights into British law. It also requires public authorities including the NHS to comply with convention rights.
- Convention rights may be absolute, limited or qualified, and give rise to positive and negative obligations.
- The right to life prohibits intentional deprivation of life, but allows the withholding of life-sustaining treatment. The right to freedom from torture, inhuman or degrading treatment prohibits interventions causing unnecessary distress or loss of dignity. The right to respect for private and family life requires respect for a person's autonomy and dignity.
- Disability is defined by the Disability Discrimination Act (DDA) 1995 as a physical or mental impairment that has a substantial and long-term adverse effect on a person's ability to carry out normal day-to-day activities.
- Discrimination under the DDA 1995 occurs when a person is treated less favourably because of their disability and that treatment cannot be justified.
- Discrimination on the grounds of race was outlawed by the Race Relations Act 1976. The Race Relations Amendment Act 2000 imposes a positive obligation on public bodies, including the NHS, to promote race equality in all areas of their work.
- The Equality Act 2010 brings anti-discriminatory legislation under one modern piece of legislation.
- The Equality and Human Rights Commission has extensive legal powers and is able to take legal action on behalf of individuals.

Knowledge review

Having completed the chapter, how would you now rate your knowledge of the following topics?

	Good	Adequate	Poor
1. Rights and obligations in healthcare.			
2. The impact of the Human Rights Act 1998 on healthcare.			
3. The law protecting women from discrimination.			
4. The role of the Equality and Human Rights Commission.			

Where you're not confident in your knowledge of a topic, what will you do next?

Activities: brief outline answers

Activity 4.1: Research and group work (page 52)

You might select article 8 as being relevant to midwifery because women have a right to respect for a private and family life. For example, it would be a breach of article 8 if a baby immediately after birth was placed into public care without considering alternatives (*K & T v Finland [2000]*).

Further reading

For a broader discussion on health and human rights we recommend:

Annas, G, Marks, S, Gruskin, S and Grodin, M (2004) *Perspectives on Health and Human Rights*. London: Routledge.

A more focused discussion of human rights and disability can be found in:

Clements, L and Read, J (2007) *Disabled People and the Right to Life: The protection and violation of disabled people's most basic human rights*. London: Routledge.

Shakespeare, T (2006) *Disability Rights and Wrongs*. London: Routledge.

For a broader discussion on diversity in healthcare we recommend:

Spector, R (2008) *Cultural Diversity in Health and Illness*, 6th edn. London: Prentice Hall.

Useful websites

www.dh.gov.uk/en/Managingyourorganisation/Equalityandhumanrights/index.htm The government's guidance on equality, diversity and human rights in healthcare.

www.echr.coe.int/ECHR/EN/Header/Case-Law/HUDOC/HUDOC+database Up-to-date judgments from the European Court of Human Rights.

www.equalityhumanrights.com Equality and Human Rights Commission, for more general cases of discrimination advice and support.

www.nhsla.com/HumanRights The National Health Service Litigation Authority maintains a human rights information service with newsletters and case sheets.

www.opsi.gov.uk/ACTS/acts1998/ukpga_19980042_en_1 A full copy of the Human Rights Act 1998 can be found here.

Chapter 5

Consent to examination and treatment

Introduction

Following on from the discussion of autonomy in Chapter 2 and human rights in Chapter 4, this chapter examines the legal expression of those rights and principles through the law relating to consent and its particular relevance to midwifery. It begins with an exploration of the extent of autonomy and role of consent, then moves on to consider specific issues such as free birthing and the refusal of caesarean sections. The chapter takes you through the process of obtaining consent before introducing the key concept of decision-making capacity and how the provisions of the Mental Capacity Act 2005 set out the requirements for assessing capacity and making decisions for those women who are unable to make care and treatment decisions for themselves.

Midwifery is a 'hands on', interactive profession. Midwives have a duty to diagnose pregnancy, and to assess and monitor women holistically throughout the pre-conception, antenatal, intrapartum and postnatal periods. This requires physical examination, care and treatment that generally require consent.

The right to self-determination

The right to touch an individual is limited in law and there is an initial presumption that it must not occur without permission.

The law recognises that adults have a right to determine what will be done to their bodies (*Schloendroff v Society of New York Hospitals* (1914)). Touching a person without consent is generally unlawful and will amount to a trespass to the person or, more rarely, a criminal assault.

Bodily integrity is held in very high regard by the law. Unlike other civil wrongs, such as negligence (see Chapter 10), any unlawful touching is actionable even if done with the best of motives. As Baroness Elizabeth Butler-Sloss stated in *Re MB (Caesarean Section)* [1997] (CA):

> The right to determine what shall be done with one's own body is a fundamental right in our society. The concepts inherent in this right are the bedrock upon which the principles of self-determination and individual autonomy are based. Free individual choice in matters affecting this right should, in my opinion, be accorded very high priority.

This fundamental principle is reflected in a midwife's professional obligations as well as in law. The NMC's *Code* (2008a) requires you to:

- ensure that you gain consent before you begin any treatment or care;
- respect and support people's rights to accept or decline treatment and care;
- uphold people's rights to be fully involved in decisions about their care;
- be aware of the legislation regarding mental capacity, ensuring that people who lack capacity remain at the centre of decision making and are fully safeguarded;
- be able to demonstrate that you have acted in someone's best interests if you have provided care in an emergency.

The obligations on a midwife imposed by the *Code* and Baroness Butler-Sloss's comments highlight the high regard in which the profession and the law holds the right to self-determination by protecting individuals from violations of bodily integrity. It is not appropriate for midwives to act paternalistically or impose their values and beliefs on the mother – even if society would consider the woman's views to be abhorrent.

CASE STUDY: Refusal of caesarean section

In *St George's Healthcare NHS Trust v S* [1998], a woman 36 weeks into her pregnancy was diagnosed with pre-eclampsia and advised of the severity of the risk to her health, and that of the unborn child, unless she was admitted to hospital for urgent medical treatment. When the woman rejected that advice she was detained for assessment under the Mental Health Act 1983 and then transferred to another hospital where, despite her continued refusal to consent to treatment, she had a caesarean section. She was then returned to the mental hospital and her detention was terminated. The woman went to court arguing that her treatment was unlawful.

The court agreed that her treatment was unlawful and held that, irrespective of the risks to her own life, a woman of sound mind had the right to refuse medical treatment. Where that woman was pregnant, the unborn child's need for medical help did not override the mother's right to refuse invasive treatment, however repugnant her decision might seem in moral terms.

The Mental Health Act 1983 cannot be used to bring about the detention of someone against her will just because her thinking might seem unusual, irrational or contrary to public opinion. Unless her capacity to consent is reduced, the person retains the right to withhold consent to medical procedures unrelated to any mental condition.

The propriety of treatment

Consent goes further than merely a defence to a claim of trespass to the person. It goes to the very heart of the propriety of treatment.

In *Airedale NHS Trust v Bland* [1993], Lord Mustill considered:

> Any invasion of the body of one person by another is potentially both a crime and a tort. How is it that [midwives] can with immunity perform on a consenting woman an act which would be a very serious crime if done by someone else?
>
> The answer must be that bodily invasions in the course of proper examination and treatment stand completely outside the criminal law. The reason why the consent is so important is not that it furnishes a defence in itself but because it is usually essential to the propriety of medical treatment.
>
> If the consent is absent, and is not dispensed with in special circumstances by operation of law, the acts of [the midwife] lose their immunity.

Lord Mustill suggests that the very rightness of an examination or treatment is underpinned by the woman's consent. This is particularly the case where the touching is to a sensitive or intimate part of the body.

CASE STUDY: Indecent assault

In *R v Ghosh* [1999], a doctor was convicted on two counts of indecent assault on a female patient. The doctor had handled her breasts on one occasion, and on a later occasion handled her breasts and inserted a finger into her anus and her vagina.

CASE STUDY *continued*

The court held that the doctor's behaviour lacked propriety and so his acts did not amount to proper treatment. He was sentenced to three years' imprisonment for indecent assault.

The quality of consent

As well as requiring midwives to restrict their touching of patients to that required in the course of proper treatment, the law also demands that the quality of consent reflects the sensitive nature of the intimate procedure.

When giving consent for such a procedure, patients are entitled to expect that the midwife is qualified to carry it out. In *R v Tabassum* [2000], a man examined the breasts of three women after they consented to participate in a survey he said he was doing in relation to breast cancer. All the women assumed the man was medically qualified in some way as he wore a white coat, but he was not. When the women discovered this they complained to the police. The man argued that he had only touched the women in the way they had consented to and that he had no sexual motive. The Court of Appeal held that sexual motive was irrelevant. For intimate examinations patients were entitled to a person who was qualified to carry out the procedure. As *Tabassum* was not medically qualified in any way, the necessary quality of the consent was absent and so the consent was not valid. *Tabassum* was sentenced to two years' imprisonment for indecent assault.

Intimate examinations and treatment therefore require that:

- a suitably qualified or supervised person undertakes the procedure;
- the consent of the patient is obtained before the procedure;
- the procedure is deemed to be proper treatment.

Where any of those conditions are not met, the actions of the midwife lose their immunity and both criminal and civil liability might arise.

Chaperones

Further protection for the midwife and patient against allegations of wrongdoing may be provided by the use of a chaperone.

Activity 5.1   *Reflection*

It is not uncommon for a midwife to be asked to act as a chaperone for a woman.

- Write down what you consider to be the role of the chaperone.
- Who do you think should fulfil that role in healthcare?

Read on for further information on this activity.

The role of chaperone for intimate examinations and treatments was considered by the *Independent Investigation Into How The NHS Handled Allegations About the Conduct of Clifford Ayling* (DH, 2004), where a doctor was convicted of 12 counts of indecent assault on his female patients.

The inquiry found no common definition of the role of a chaperone (DH, 2004, para. 2.51), but four differing definitions were considered.

- A chaperone provides a safeguard for a patient against humiliation, pain or distress during an examination and protects against verbal, physical, sexual or other abuse.
- A chaperone provides physical and emotional comfort and reassurance to a patient during sensitive and intimate examinations or treatment.
- An experienced chaperone will identify unusual or unacceptable behaviour on the part of the healthcare professional.
- A chaperone may also provide protection for the healthcare professional from potentially abusive patients.

A chaperone's role may be passive (as a simple witness to the examination), or active (as a participant in the procedure, providing comfort and reassurance and being skilled in identifying unacceptable behaviour).

The Ayling Inquiry (DH, 2004, paras 2.58–2.60) recommended that:

- each NHS Trust and Health Board has a chaperoning policy and makes this explicit to patients and resources it accordingly;
- there must be accredited training for the role and an identified managerial lead with responsibility for the implementation of the policy;
- any reported breaches of the chaperoning policy must be formally investigated and treated, if deliberate, as a disciplinary matter;
- best practice demands that the chaperone policy must ensure that:
  - no family member or friend of a patient should be expected to undertake any formal chaperoning role;
  - the presence of a chaperone during a clinical examination and treatment must be the clearly expressed choice of a patient;
  - the woman has the right to decline any chaperone offered if she so wishes;
  - chaperoning should not be undertaken by other than trained staff: the use of untrained administrative staff as chaperones is not acceptable.

Elements of a valid consent

To be a valid defence to a claim of trespass, consent needs to satisfy three key elements. It must be:

- full;
- freely given;
- reasonably informed.

Full consent

When obtaining consent you must ensure that the woman agrees to all the treatment you intend to carry out. Proceeding with treatment that the patient is unaware of, or has refused to agree to, will be a trespass to the person and actionable in law (*Williamson v East London & City HA* [1998]). You must therefore take care to explain all the treatment or touching that will occur when obtaining consent from a woman, and ensure that additional treatment or touching is subject to further consent.

CASE STUDY: Examination without consent

A midwife faced a competence and conduct committee of the NMC when she tried to carry out an intimate examination without consent (*Lancashire Telegraph*, 2009). The committee heard that the midwife tried to examine the expectant mother without her permission, despite the woman's cries of protest and attempts to push her away.

She was found guilty of professional misconduct and her name was removed from the register.

Freely given consent

Consent is an expression of autonomy and so must be the free choice of the individual. It cannot be obtained by threat, force or undue influence. This does not mean that a midwife cannot influence a woman's decision. Indeed, part of your role is to explain the benefits of treatment and care in order to obtain consent.

In law, undue influence must erode the individual's free will. It must be so forceful that all other considerations are excluded when making a choice, such as where a threat of force or harm forces a woman to accept or refuse treatment.

CASE STUDY: No undue influence

In *Centre for Reproductive Medicine v U* [2002], a widow appealed against a decision permitting the destruction of her late husband's sperm, which had been surgically removed and stored. Prior to the sperm being removed, he had signed a consent form in which he had agreed that the sperm could be used after his death. He later withdrew this aspect of his consent at the request of a specialist nursing sister when it was explained that use after death caused ethical problems.

Mrs U contended that her husband had withdrawn his consent reluctantly and only because he believed that, if he did not, treatment would cease or be postponed. She argued that he had been unduly influenced by the nurse. The court found that Mr U's withdrawal of his consent to the posthumous storage and use of his sperm had not been due to undue influence. The nurse had influenced his decision by explaining the difficulty of allowing the posthumous use of sperm, but she had not unduly influenced him. Mr U had listened to the nurse, asked questions, weighed his options and arrived at a freely given decision.

Undue influence may also be brought to bear by family members. Midwives must be certain that the choice being made is that of the woman and is not due to the outside influence of family members.

CASE STUDY: Refusal of treatment

In *Re T (Adult: Refusal of Treatment)* [1992], a woman who initially consented to a caesarean section changed her mind following a visit from her mother, a person with strong views on the use of blood, and would only proceed without blood products. When *Miss T* later required a blood transfusion, the court held that her refusal of treatment had been negatived by the undue influence of her mother, her refusal of treatment was not freely given and so the transfusion could proceed.

Reasonably informed consent

The law is clear that part of a midwife's duty is to give advice and information to a woman so that she understands the nature of the treatment proposed and can make a choice (*Hills v Potter* [1983]). The courts do not distinguish between advice given in a therapeutic and non-therapeutic context, such as when a midwife gives contraceptive advice (*Gold v Haringey HA* [1987]).

The basis of the duty to give information is derived from two areas of law: the law of trespass and the law of negligence (see Chapter 10).

Trespass to the person

In trespass a real or effective consent requires the midwife to explain in broad terms the nature of the treatment to the woman. As long as the broad nature of the touching has been explained, no cause of action in trespass will arise.

CASE STUDY: Misinformation

In *Potts v NWRHA* (1983), a patient successfully sued for battery when she was led to believe that she was having a routine postnatal vaccination. In fact, she was given the long-acting contraceptive Depo-provera. If a midwife gives misinformation or false information to a patient, consent will be negatived and liability in trespass will arise.

Negligence

The second type of information required to be given to a patient concerns the risks of having treatment. Here, the courts have been quick to point out that a failure to disclose risks does not vitiate a real consent and no action is possible in trespass (*Hills v Potter* [1983]). The proper cause of action in disclosure of risks cases falls in negligence.

Breach in the standard of care

Midwives owe a duty to take reasonable care not to cause harm to the women they are attending. They are required to give advice and information to the standard of the ordinary midwife (*Bolam v Friern HMC* [1957]). This is called the *Bolam* test and is judged by reference to what information a respected body of midwives would have given in the same circumstances. However, be mindful that the court can reject a practice if it does not stand up to logical analysis (*Bolitho v City & Hackney HA* [1997]).

Activity 5.2   Reflection

- How much information do you think women should be given about their treatment?
- Should they be told every last detail or just what you consider important?
- Should a woman who asks questions be told more than one who is content to listen to your advice without asking questions?

As the answer depends on your own views and experience, there is no outline answer at the end of the chapter.

Guidance on giving information in particular circumstances has been set out by the courts. You would do well to inform your practice by reference to this guidance.

How much information to disclose

The issue of how much information a person should receive about risks was considered by the House of Lords in *Sidaway v Bethlem Royal Hospital* [1985], where the court decided that, as a general rule, the amount of information to be given must be based on the standard of care in *Bolam*. Midwives must ensure that sufficient information is given to enable the woman to make a choice.

This requires that midwives disclose material risks, but withhold information if a woman would be frightened if told all risks and the likelihood of occurrence was very small.

CASE STUDY: *Failure to tell*

In *Goorkani v Tayside Health Board* [1991], a doctor was found negligent for failing to tell a patient of the risk of irreversible infertility at the time of prescribing chlorambucil for Behcet's disease. The risk of infertility when used over the longer term rose to 95 per cent and this transpired in Mr Goorkani's case.

No therapeutic lying

The notion of lying to a person to calm them before treatment was considered in *Hatcher v Black* [1954], where a singer claimed damages for negligence when an operation resulted in her left vocal cord being paralysed even though she had been told there was no risk. The judge appeared to condone a form of therapeutic lying when he said that, on the evening before the operation, the singer was told that there was no risk to her voice even though there was some slight risk. She was told a lie, but in the circumstances it was justifiable.

In the *Sidaway* case, the House of Lords rejected therapeutic lying. They stressed that, while information may be withheld, the midwife's duty was to answer as truthfully and fully as the question required. Lying about risks to calm a woman would be a breach of duty.

When giving information about the material risks inherent in treatment, a midwife's answer would depend on:

- the circumstances;
- the nature of the enquiry;
- the nature of the information that is available;
- the reliability of the information;
- the relevance of the information and the condition of the patient.

Specific questions about specific risks

A different test applies to women who ask specific questions about the risk of treatment. In *Chester v Afshar* [2002], the Court of Appeal held that, when responding to specific questioning about risks, the midwife is required to answer fully and truthfully regardless of the likelihood of the risk materialising. In *Chester*, the risk of nerve root damage was estimated at less than 1 per cent. However, as the patient had specifically asked about such risks and had not been given adequate advice, the doctor was found to be negligent as he had not given a full and honest answer.

Duty to inform of mishap

Where a mishap occurs during treatment, the midwife's duty of care requires that the woman is informed of the mishap immediately. In *Gerber v Pines* (1935), a doctor was giving an injection when the needle broke due to a muscle spasm. He did not tell the woman what had happened until he arranged for it to be removed surgically a week later. The court held that, although the injection was not negligently given, there was a breach of duty by the doctor in not informing the woman immediately of the mishap.

Should a mishap occur during treatment the midwife must inform the woman immediately.

Obtaining consent

Activity 5.3   *Reflection*

Note down the methods you have used to obtain consent from the women you have examined.

- What is the most common form of consent you use?

As the answer depends on your own views and experience, there is no outline answer at the end of the chapter.

Consent may be obtained in two ways. A woman may express her consent. That is, she makes known her willingness to be touched. Express consent can be written or oral. Written consent is usually obtained where a procedure is invasive, such as surgery, or perceived to carry a material risk, such as an immunisation, and is often taken by means of a consent form.

This provides a degree of evidential certainty that the woman agreed to treatment. It must not be relied on too heavily, however. Lord Donaldson, in *Re T (Adult: Refusal of Treatment)* [1992], pointed out that a consent form was only as useful as the understanding of the person signing it. When obtaining consent, whether in writing or orally, it is essential that an explanation of treatment and other material facts must be recorded in your records to corroborate the consent.

The second form of consent is an implied consent. This is permission implied through the actions of the woman in response to a request to provide treatment. An obvious example would be a woman holding out an arm and rolling up a sleeve when you ask for permission to take her blood pressure. Implied consent does not mean, however, that agreeing to come to hospital or allowing a midwife into the home implies agreement to treatment. Every episode of care or treatment must be subject to a valid consent.

Evidential certainty

As a matter of law each form of consent, whether it is verbal, written or implied, is equally effective and it does not matter which method you use. From an evidential perspective it is clear that a written consent provides evidence that consent was obtained. Whichever method you use to obtain consent it is essential that your contemporaneous entry in your records corroborates that consent was given and that the woman was happy to proceed with treatment.

Withdrawing consent

Consent is a continuous process and may be withdrawn at any time. A withdrawal of consent is indistinguishable from an initial refusal to consent. Midwives must accept that, if a woman changes her mind and refuses to continue with treatment, it must cease or trespass to the person will occur.

CASE STUDY: Consent has to be renewed

In *Ciarlariello v Schacter* [1991], a woman underwent a cerebral angiogram before which the doctor explained the effects and risks of the procedure. During the course of a second angiogram she became agitated and insisted that the procedure be stopped.

Later she agreed to the procedure continuing, during which she suffered a stroke and was paralysed. She sued, arguing that she would not have agreed to carry on if she had been reminded of the risks.

The right to decide on treatment

In *Re T (Adult: Refusal of Treatment)* [1992], the Court of Appeal held that the right to decide presupposes an ability or a capacity to do so. Decision-making capacity is the key to autonomy. If a woman has capacity, her decisions are binding on you. An adult woman with decision-making capacity has the right to accept or refuse treatment even if doing so will lead to her death. This reflects the fundamental respect for autonomy in healthcare. It is not for you to judge a capable patient's decision on treatment against your values.

CASE STUDY: Entitlement to refuse treatment

A 22-year-old mother died just hours after giving birth to twins because doctors were forbidden from giving her a blood transfusion as she was a Jehovah's Witness (Attewill, 2007).

Complications set in after the birth that required an immediate emergency transfusion. Although the care team explained the consequences of not having treatment, the patient refused the blood due to her religious beliefs.

As a capable adult patient she was entitled to refuse the blood, and the care team was required in law to accept her decision even though the consequences were that she died.

Free birthing

Free birthing occurs where a woman decides to give birth without medical or professional help. The popularity of the practice is growing. Free birthing is lawful as long as the birth is not attended by an unqualified person. This unqualified person may be a non-registered midwife, doula, nurse, the partner, relative or a friend who is not a registered midwife or registered doctor. Under the provisions of the Nursing and Midwifery Order 2001, part 9, articles 44 and 45, it is unlawful for an unqualified person to undertake the role of a registered midwife or attend a woman in childbirth unless in an emergency or in supported recognised training. In free birthing the woman assumes responsibility for her birth, but can have her partner, relative or friend present in a supportive role only.

A midwife has no right to be at a baby's birth if a woman chooses to exercise her autonomy by not contacting or engaging a midwife.

CASE STUDY: Husband charged with manslaughter

In *R v Smith* [1979], Smith's wife had a marked aversion to doctors and medical treatment. When she went into labour at home she refused to allow her husband to call for any form of assistance. Sadly, her child was stillborn and the body was hidden in a cupboard. She continued to feel unwell and, although Smith wanted to call a doctor, his wife would not let him and she died. Smith was charged with her manslaughter. The judge directed the jury that, as his wife was an adult with decision-making capacity, she could remove him of his duty to seek medical attention for her by refusing to have such attention. Smith's wife had exercised her right to refuse to be attended at the birth and to refuse medical care after the birth and Smith could not therefore be guilty of manslaughter.

The NMC (2008b) requires midwives to respect a woman's choice for unassisted birthing, be empathetic, adhere to the NMC's *Code* and the *Midwives Rules and Standards*, and not be critical of this choice or outcome. If a midwife is concerned with a mother's physical or psychological well-being, decision-making capacity or safety, he or she must inform their manager and SoM immediately.

Decision-making capacity

Decision-making capacity is the ability to make a decision and it is the key to autonomy (*Re T (Adult: Refusal of Treatment)* [1992]). It is based on a person understanding and using information about treatment when making a decision.

Decision-making capacity can vary over time and can depend on the decision to be made. A woman might have the requisite capacity to make a simple decision but not the requisite capacity to make a complex decision. Capacity is based on a test of understanding and is not a professional or status test. You cannot assume lack of capacity because of a woman's age, physical appearance, condition or an aspect of her behaviour.

Mental Capacity Act 2005

Women aged 16 and over are assumed in law to have the ability to make decisions about their pregnancy and maternity care and their consent to treatment is required before it can proceed.

Where a woman lacks decision-making capacity, the Mental Capacity Act 2005 and its guiding principles ensure that their rights and interests are at the centre of the decision-making process.

Concept summary: The principles of the Mental Capacity Act 2005

- A person must be assumed to have capacity unless it is established that he or she lacks capacity.
- A person is not to be treated as unable to make a decision unless all practicable steps to help him or her to do so have been taken without success.
- A person is not to be treated as unable to make a decision merely because he or she makes an unwise decision.
- An act done, or decision made, under this Act for or on behalf of a person who lacks capacity must be done, or made, in his or her best interests.
- Before the act is done, or the decision is made, regard must be had to whether the purpose for which it is needed can be as effectively achieved in a way that is less restrictive of the person's rights and freedom of action.

The Mental Capacity Act 2005 requires you to assume that a woman aged 16 or older has the capacity to make decisions, even unwise decisions, for herself. You are able to act on that decision to accept or refuse treatment without the need to assess decision-making capacity. The need to assess capacity only arises where the behaviour or circumstances of the woman triggers a doubt in your mind about her ability to make a decision. The principle stresses a woman's right to autonomy and is further supported by requiring steps to be taken to maximise decision-making capacity.

Activity 5.4   **Group work**

The law recognises that some women may require support to make decisions.

- In a group, discuss what practicable steps you could take to help a woman make a decision about her care and treatment.

Read on for further information.

The code of practice to the Mental Capacity Act 2005 (Department for Constitutional Affairs, 2007) suggests that practical steps might include:

- using simple language and, where appropriate, pictures and objects rather than words;
- arranging for the person to have the information in their preferred language;
- consulting whoever knows the person well on the best methods of communication;
- choosing the best time and location where the person feels at ease;
- waiting until the person's capacity improves before requiring a decision.

Where a woman is considered to lack decision-making capacity, any action or decision taken must be in their best interests.

The final guiding principle of the Mental Capacity Act 2005 requires you to act in the least restrictive way possible. This important requirement will ensure that any interference with a person's rights and freedom to make decisions will be limited to that required to meet the immediate needs of the individual.

CASE STUDY: Best interests

In *Re S (Adult Patient: Sterilisation: Patient's Best Interests)* [2001], the mother of a woman aged 29 and born with severe learning difficulties was concerned about the possibility of her becoming pregnant when she moved into a home, and applied for a sterilisation on her behalf.

The court refused, saying that it was in the woman's best interests to allow the insertion of an intrauterine device as it was the least invasive option, was not irreversible, and left room for surgical procedures if it proved to be ineffective.

Assessing decision-making capacity

A woman lacks capacity where an impairment or disturbance of the mind or brain affects her ability to make a particular decision. It does not matter whether the lack of capacity is permanent or temporary.

CASE STUDY: Capacity affected by phobia

In *Re MB* [1997], following a medical examination MB (who was pregnant) was informed that a caesarean delivery might be required. She consented to the operation but then refused to be given anaesthesia by injection because she had a severe phobia of needles.

The court found that a person did not have capacity where an impairment of mental functioning made them unable to decide whether consent should be given, and temporary factors, including panic brought on by fear, could completely erode capacity.

MB temporarily lacked capacity because of her fear of needles and, therefore, the doctors were entitled to administer the anaesthetic in an emergency because it was in her best interests to do so.

The test for decision-making capacity is a two-stage functional test based on the decision to be made at that time, rather than a general ability to make decisions. That is, the following questions must be asked.

- Is there a permanent or temporary impairment or disturbance to the functioning of the mind or brain?
- If there is, how far is it affecting the person's ability to make a decision?

A woman will not be capable of making a decision if, due to an impairment or disturbance to the mind or brain, she is unable to:

- understand the treatment information relevant to the decision; or
- retain the information long enough to make a decision; or
- use or weigh the information as part of the process of arriving at a decision; or
- communicate that decision by any means.

It will generally be for you to determine whether the woman you are providing treatment to has decision-making capacity. Where the situation is more serious, many other people become involved in the care and treatment. It is then the person in charge, usually the senior doctor, who will determine if the woman has decision-making capacity. If a dispute over capacity remains unresolved, the courts can make the determination.

Stages of the assessment process

- **The trigger phase**
  - You must assume that a woman 16 years or older has capacity to consent to care or treatment unless a concern triggers a doubt in your mind.
- **The practical support phase**
  - You cannot say a woman lacks decision-making capacity unless you have taken practical steps to help them to make a decision.
- **The diagnostic threshold**
  - Are you able to discern an impairment or disturbance to the functioning of the person's mind or brain? It does not matter if this is permanent or temporary. If you cannot determine such an impairment or disturbance, no further action can be taken under the Mental Capacity Act 2005.
- **The assessment phase**
  - How far is the impairment or disturbance to the mind or brain affecting the ability to make a decision?
  - Where a woman cannot
    - understand treatment information; or
    - retain treatment information; or
    - use or weigh treatment information when making a decision; or
    - communicate their decision in some way;
    - you can reasonably conclude that she lacks capacity for that particular decision.

CASE STUDY: Denial

In *Norfolk and Norwich Healthcare NHS Trust v W* [1997], W, who had a history of mental health problems, arrived at hospital ready to deliver her baby but in a state of arrested labour and denying that she was pregnant. She would not consent to the caesarean that was urgently needed.

The court authorised treatment because W lacked the decision-making capacity to make the decision because she was incapable of weighing up the considerations involved.

Designated decision makers

The Mental Capacity Act 2005 has two formal powers that allow a third party to make decisions on behalf of a woman who lacks decision-making capacity. These powers can give the designated decision maker the right to consent to or refuse medical treatment. Where a designated decision maker with authority is in place, his or her consent must be obtained before care and treatment can lawfully be given.

Health and welfare lasting powers of attorney

A power allowing another to consent on behalf of a person who lacks capacity can be created through a health and welfare lasting power of attorney (LPA). The LPA must be created by the person (the donor) when they are capable and can only come into force when the person lacks capacity and the LPA has been registered with the Office of Public Guardian.

A person can also create an LPA that allows another to manage their property and affairs.

Court of Protection deputy

When continuing decisions need to be made on behalf of a person who lacks capacity and there is no LPA, the Court of Protection may appoint a deputy to make health and welfare decisions on the person's behalf that can include the right to consent to or refuse treatment.

The Court must be satisfied that the deputy is willing and able to fulfil the role and that appointing a deputy is a proportionate response to the needs of the patient.

Advance decisions refusing treatment

As well as having designated decision makers able to make consent to treatment decisions, a person can make an advance decision to refuse treatment. Where a valid applicable advance refusal is in place, the wishes of the person must be respected and treatment withheld. Only compulsory treatment for mental disorder, other than electro-convulsive therapy (ECT), under the Mental Health Act 1983, can override a valid and applicable advance decision refusing healthcare.

Although an advance decision can be made orally, where it is to apply to life-sustaining treatment, the Mental Capacity Act 2005, section 25, requires that it is:

- made in writing;
- signed by the person or signed on their behalf in their presence;
- witnessed in writing in the presence of the person;
- verified by a statement made by the maker that expressly and specifically states that the advanced decision is to apply even if life is at risk.

Best interests

The Mental Capacity Act 2005 provides a checklist of factors that must be considered when determining whether care and treatment is in the best interests of a person who lacks capacity. This holistic approach to best interests ensures that the wishes of the person and views of those caring for him or her are taken into account.

When determining whether care and treatment is in an incapable patient's best interests, you must:

- consider all the relevant circumstances;
- consider whether the decision can wait until the person regains capacity;
- as far as reasonably practicable, permit and encourage the person to participate in their care and treatment;
- not be motivated by a desire to bring about the death of the patient;
- consider, so far as is reasonably ascertainable:
  - the person's past and present wishes and feelings (and, in particular, any relevant written statement made when they had capacity);
  - the beliefs and values that would be likely to influence their decision if they had capacity;
  - other factors that they would be likely to consider if they were able to do so;
  - take into account, if it is practicable and appropriate to consult them, the views of:
  - anyone named by the person as someone to be consulted on the matter in question or on matters of that kind;
  - anyone engaged in caring for the person or interested in his or her welfare;

- any donee of an LPA granted by the person;
- any deputy appointed for the person by the court.

Independent Mental Capacity Advocate

Where no suitable person is available to be consulted on what would be in the best interests of a person who lacks decision-making capacity, there may be a duty to instruct an Independent Mental Capacity Advocate (IMCA). The IMCA will make representations about the person's wishes, feelings and beliefs and call the decision-maker's attention to the factors relevant to their decision.

An IMCA will only be involved where the decision concerns:

- serious medical treatment; that is, treatment that involves providing, withdrawing or withholding treatment in circumstances where:
  - in a case where a single treatment is being proposed, there is a fine balance between its benefits to the patient and the burdens and risks it is likely to entail for him or her;
  - in a case where there is a choice of treatments, a decision as to which one to use is finely balanced; or
  - what is proposed would be likely to involve serious consequences for the patient.
  - a change in the person's accommodation where it is provided by the NHS or local authority; or
  - authorised detention under the deprivation of liberty safeguards.

Protection from liability

Where care and treatment for an incapable adult proceeds following an assessment of capacity and determination of best interests, the care giver is protected from liability in the law relating to consent.

Restraint

Restraint is defined as:

> the use or threat of force where the person is resisting and any restriction of liberty of movement whether or not the person resists.

This wide definition includes even mild forms of restraint, such as holding an incapable person's arm to keep it still when taking a blood sample. Restraint is permitted, but only if it is proportionate and only when the person using it reasonably believes it is necessary to prevent harm to the incapable person.

Court of Protection

The Court of Protection is a specialist court that hears cases and settles matters concerning people who lack capacity. The Court can also appoint deputies (see page 88) and give them powers to make ongoing decisions for incapable adults.

Office of the Public Guardian

The Office of the Public Guardian is responsible for the supervision of deputies appointed by the Court of Protection and for supporting deputies in their role. It also has a role in protecting people subject to the Court's powers from abuse or exploitation by:

- keeping a register of LPAs;
- keeping a register of orders appointing deputies;

- supervising deputies appointed by the Court;
- receiving reports from attorneys;
- dealing with enquiries and complaints about deputies or attorneys.

C H A P T E R   S U M M A R Y

- The moral principle of autonomy is given its legal expression in the law relating to consent.
- Consent is essential to the propriety of care and treatment.
- A legally valid consent will protect the practitioner from the tort of trespass to the person and the criminal offence of assault and battery.
- A valid consent must be full, free from duress and reasonably informed.
- An adult with decision-making capacity is able to refuse treatment even if such refusal might lead to his or her death.
- Where there is doubt about the capacity of a person 16 or older to make a treatment decision, their capacity must be assessed in accordance with the guiding principles of the Mental Capacity Act 2005.
- Treatment for a person who lacks capacity can only proceed if it is in their best interests.
- Best interests must be determined in accordance with the checklist of factors set out under the Mental Capacity Act 2005.
- Where a person appears to lack decision-making capacity, the provisions of the Mental Capacity Act 2005 and its code of practice set out the requirements for assessing capacity and determining what care and treatment is in the person's best interests. It also allows for designated decision makers to consent to treatment for people who lack capacity.
- These arrangements are overseen by the Court of Protection and the Office of the Public Guardian.

Knowledge review

Having completed the chapter, how would you now rate your knowledge of the following topics?

	Good	Adequate	Poor
1. The relationship between the ethical principle of autonomy and the law of trespass to the person.			
2. The role of consent in healthcare.			
3. The elements of a valid consent.			
4. Decision-making capacity.			
5. The provisions for providing care and treatment to a person who lacks decision-making capacity.			

Where you're not confident in your knowledge of a topic, what will you do next?

Further reading

Department for Constitutional Affairs (2007) *Mental Capacity Act 2005 Code of Practice*. London: The Stationery Office.
Department of Health (DH) (2001) *Good Practice in Consent (HSC 2001/023)*. London: The Stationery Office.

Useful websites

www.dh.gov.uk The Department of Health provides a good range of information on consent, including model consent forms.
www.justice.gov.uk The Ministry of Justice site includes detailed legal guidance on the Mental Capacity Act 2005.

Chapter 6

Consent: children and infants

NMC Standards for Pre-registration Midwifery Education

This chapter will address the following competencies:

Domain: Effective midwifery practice
- Examine and care for babies immediately following birth.
- Work in partnership with women and other care providers during the postnatal period to provide seamless care and interventions.

Domain: Professional and ethical practice
- Practise in accordance with *The Code: Standards of conduct, performance and ethics for nurses and midwives* (NMC, 2008a), within the limitations of the individual's own competence, knowledge and sphere of professional practice, consistent with the legislation relating to midwifery practice.

Chapter aims

After reading this chapter, you will be able to:

- state the three developmental stages a minor child passes through to become an autonomous adult;
- outline who has parental responsibility for a baby;
- describe the extent of a person with parental responsibility's right to consent to treatment for a baby;
- apply the rule in *Gillick* when obtaining consent from mothers who are under 16 years of age;
- examine the requirements for a valid consent from a mother who is 16 or 17 years old;
- judge when it is lawful to restrict a child's liberty in order to provide maternity care and treatment.

Introduction

This chapter considers how the law of consent applies to babies and to mothers who are under 18 years old. It points out that, in the eyes of the law, a minor (a child under 18 years) moves through three developmental stages on the path to becoming an autonomous adult. Infants and young children rely on a person with parental responsibility to consent for them. This chapter outlines the people who have parental responsibility, and the extent and limits of their decision-making authority. The chapter goes on to consider how a midwife would assess a mother who was under 16 for competence to consent using the rule in *Gillick*, which allows a sufficiently mature child to make her own consent decisions. The right of mothers aged 16 and 17 to consent to treatment is considered. The chapter concludes with some dilemmas: what to do when a parent disagrees with the treatment their baby should receive, or when a young mother refuses to stay in hospital for treatment?

The child as mother

The UK has one of the highest rates of teenage pregnancy in the developed world. According to the latest available statistics, there were 42,900 teenage pregnancies in England and Wales in 2007, with 8,200 of those relating to girls under 16. Therefore, it is inevitable that you will encounter an expectant mother who is under 18 years of age, and it is essential that you are familiar with the legal and professional requirements for consent that relate to young mothers (DH/DCSF, 2009).

The nature of consent

Consent is a state of mind in which a woman agrees to the touching of her body as part of an examination or for treatment (*Sidaway v Bethlem Royal Hospital* [1985]). Consent has a clinical and legal purpose. The clinical purpose recognises that the success of treatment depends very often on the cooperation of the woman. The legal purpose is to underpin the propriety of the treatment and furnish a defence to the crime and tort of trespass (see Chapter 5). For capable adult women, the law recognises the right to self-determination, which includes the right to consent to or refuse medical treatment even if this would lead to a woman's death or the death of the unborn child.

Children reach the age of majority or adulthood at 18. However, while the courts acknowledge that no minor under 18 is wholly autonomous, they do recognise a child's right to consent to medical treatment as they develop and mature with age.

Kennedy and Grubb (1998) argue that minors pass through three developmental stages on the journey to becoming autonomous adults:

- the infant and child of tender years;
- the Gillick competent child;
- children 16 and 17 years old.

The infant and child of tender years

Midwives' care of the neonate must be in accordance with the requirements of the law and their professional code. *The Code* (NMC, 2008a) requires you to obtain consent before you give any care or treatment and when obtaining consent for a child. The involvement of those with parental responsibility in the consent procedure is usually necessary.

Parental responsibility

The Children Act 1989 created the concept of parental responsibility, defined as *all the rights, duties, powers, responsibility and authority which by law a parent has in relation to the child and its property* (Children Act 1989, s2). It empowers a person to make most decisions in a child's life, including consenting to medical treatment on the child's behalf.

Parental responsibility may be shared and generally decisions can be made independently. In most cases only the consent of one person with parental responsibility is needed to proceed with examination or treatment.

Activity 6.1   *Reflection*

- List all the people you think might have parental responsibility for a baby.

- From that list select the person who you think would have parental responsibility from the time the baby is born.

Please do not move on to the next part until you are ready for the answer.

Automatic parental responsibility

You are likely to encounter several categories of person who may have parental responsibility for a baby in your care. Parental responsibility is not exclusive to the parents in every case.

Parental responsibility is conferred automatically on the baby's mother and the father if he was married to the mother at the time of the birth (Children Act 1989, s2). If unmarried parents subsequently marry, the baby's father gains parental responsibility (Family Law Reform Act 1987, s1).

In recognition of the changing demographic of the family and to encourage both parents to play a full part in the upbringing of their children, the Children Act 1989 was amended in December 2003 to allow unmarried natural fathers to have parental responsibility once they become registered as the father under any of the birth registration statutes.

Acquired parental responsibility

If a father is not married to his baby's mother and did not become registered as the father after December 2003, he may still acquire parental responsibility under an agreement with the mother or by order of the court (Children Act 1989, s3). Similarly, the Children Act 1989, section 4ZA, allows parental responsibility to be acquired by a second female where she is recognised as the parent of the baby under the Human Fertilisation and Embryology Act 2008, section 43 (see Chapter 12 for details of the new rules on becoming a parent when a baby is born as a result of assisted conception).

Parental responsibility may be acquired by others such as those in possession of an emergency protection order or a care order under safeguarding children measures, but only for the duration of the order (see Chapter 7).

Step-parents

Since December 2005 a step-parent who is married to a baby's natural parent can acquire parental responsibility either by agreement with the natural parents or by order of the court (Children Act 1989, s4A).

Delegation of parental responsibility

The Children Act 1989, section 2(9), allows a person with parental responsibility to arrange for someone else to exercise it on their behalf. This delegation need not be in writing and allows carers such as schools, nannies and childminders to make delegated decisions on behalf of a person with parental responsibility for the child. For example, a midwife may visit a baby only to find her in the care of her grandmother. As long as the midwife is satisfied that the grandmother is acting with the authority of a person with parental responsibility, she may accept the grandmother's consent as permission to treat the child.

The extent of parental responsibility

Although a person with parental responsibility can generally make decisions independently, the freedom of each to act alone is not unfettered. The court held in *Re J* [2000] that there is a small group of important decisions that should not to be carried out or arranged by one parent alone, although he or she has parental responsibility under the Children Act 1989.

Activity 6.2   *Reflection*

What kind of decisions do you think should not be made by one parent alone?

Please do not move on to the next part until you are ready for the answer.

Where the agreement of each person with parental responsibility is not forthcoming, the decision must not be made without the specific approval of the court. As held in *Re B (A Child)* [2003], these important decisions include:

- sterilisation of a child;
- the change of a child's surname;
- circumcision of a child;
- a hotly disputed immunisation.

Authority to intervene

In *KD (A Minor) (Ward: Termination of Access)* [1988], the House of Lords held that the best persons to bring up a baby are the natural parents. Their view is that public authorities cannot improve on nature and parents are given the exclusive privilege of bringing up a baby with the decisions of a devoted and responsible parent being treated with respect.

However, the parent's rights exist for the benefit of the baby and must be exercised in the baby's best interests. The courts, through their inherent jurisdiction, exercise a supervisory role over parental decision making and can overrule a parental decision that is not in the best interests of the baby's welfare.

Under the private law provisions of the Children Act 1989, section 8, the courts also have the power to settle a dispute between two or more people with parental responsibility.

Private law is not a question of public protection and so the threshold criterion of significant harm does not have to be engaged for the courts to have jurisdiction.

As long as there is a dispute between people regarding an issue of parental responsibility, the courts can intervene to settle the issue.

Private law orders

The Children Act 1989, section 8, gives the courts powers to resolve disputes regarding an issue of parental responsibility. The orders available are:

- **residence order**, which settles with whom a baby should live and bestows parental responsibility on that person where necessary;
- **contact order**, which settles contact arrangements; contact can be as widely interpreted as the court sees fit and ranges from telephone and email contact to visits and holidays;
- **prohibited steps order**, prohibiting an action without the permission of the court;
- **specific issues order**, allowing the court to settle a specific issue in relation to parental responsibility.

Where the health and welfare of a baby are at issue, the courts have been prepared to use these orders in a creative way.

Scenario

A child lives with her grandmother at the request of her mother, but the grandmother finds that the GP and midwife will not accept her consent for such things as immunisations and examinations.

The grandmother goes to court, which grants her a residence order because the welfare of the baby requires her to have parental responsibility, even though where the baby lives is not an issue.

(For a real-life example of the creative use of private law orders you may wish to read *B v B (A Minor) (Residence Order)* [1992].)

Prohibited steps and specific issues orders are also used by the courts to settle issues concerning a child's healthcare. In *J (A Minor) (Prohibited Steps Order: Circumcision)* [2000], the English mother of J was granted a prohibited steps order preventing his Muslim father from making arrangements for him to be circumcised without a court order, because ritual circumcision was an irreversible operation that was not medically necessary and had physical and psychological risks, and in such cases the consent of both parents was essential.

CASE STUDY: A specific issues order

In *Camden LBC v R (A Minor) (Blood Transfusion)* [1993], a baby's parents refused to allow him to have a blood transfusion for the treatment of B-cell lymphoblastic leukaemia due to their religious beliefs. The court found that, where life was at risk, it was essential to act urgently. The private law requirements of the Children Act 1989, section 8, could be used to seek a specific issues order. This procedure allows the matter to be brought before a High Court judge, who could order the treatment without delay and without transferring parental responsibility.

Authorising treatment against the wishes of a baby's parents is reserved for the most serious cases. In *A&D v B&E* [2003], the High Court accepted that, in general, there is wide scope for parental objection to medical intervention. The Court considers medical interventions as existing on a scale. At one end are obvious cases where parental objection would have no value in welfare terms, for example urgent life-saving treatment. At the other end are cases where there is genuine scope for debate and the views of the parents are important. These would not raise questions of neglect or abuse that would trigger public protection proceedings. Although an NHS Trust can obtain leave to apply for a specific issues order (Children Act 1989, s8), it is unlikely that leave would be granted in the face of unified parental opposition to this type of treatment.

CASE STUDY: Urgent and non-urgent treatment

In *Re P (A Minor)* (1981), the court directed that a termination could proceed on a 15-year-old child despite the genuinely held objections of her parents on religious and other grounds.

In *Re B (A Child)* [2003], the Court of Appeal held that, while it was prepared to settle a dispute between two parents on the issue of childhood immunisations, it would not do so where the dispute was between a parent and the health authorities.

The best interests test

The right of a parent to exercise their right to consent to treatment for a baby is subject to them acting in the baby's best interests. The courts are also required to act in the best interests of the welfare of a baby whenever a case is brought before them. The test for best interests has developed as new cases have been brought to court for judgment.

In one of the earliest cases, the court limited its consideration of a best interest to the life expectancy of the child. In *Re B (A Minor) (Wardship: Medical Treatment)* [1981], a baby born with Down's syndrome needed urgent surgery for an intestinal blockage. The parents took the view that it would be kinder to let the baby die than to allow her to grow up as a physically and mentally disabled person. The judge held that the surgery was straightforward and that, as the baby was expected to live 20–30 years, surgery was in her best interests.

Some ten years later the court refined the determination of a best interest to include pain and suffering. In *J (A Minor) (Child in Care: Medical Treatment)* [1993], a profoundly brain-damaged baby with a very short life expectancy was not thought to be benefiting from treatment and both the parents and medical team sought an order allowing them to curtail treatment.

The court held that, even in the case of babies, it was never the case that doctors and midwives have to continue giving treatment right to the end of the baby's life. What the court called the absolutist test never applied. The denial of treatment to prolong life could only be sanctioned where it was in the best interests of the baby and the test that applied was that of the baby's best interests in those circumstances, being based on an assessment of the quality of life, the baby's future pain and its suffering in relation to the life-saving treatment.

The need to go to court

Where those with parental responsibility strongly oppose the giving or withholding of treatment by a health professional to a baby, the matter will need to be referred to the court for a decision. Failing to seek the court's approval for a plan of care in these circumstances would be a breach of the child's right to respect for a private and family life under article 8 of the European Convention on Human Rights.

CASE STUDY: The need to go to court

In *Glass v United Kingdom* [2004], a severely physically and mentally disabled baby complained (with the aid of his mother) that the UK had violated his right to physical integrity under the European Convention on Human Rights 1950, article 8.

On his readmission with respiratory failure, the hospital insisted that he was dying and that diamorphine should be given to relieve his obvious distress. His mother disagreed and objected to the proposed treatment in the belief that it would harm his chances of recovery. Despite her objection, diamorphine was administered, but his condition improved and he returned home.

The European Court of Human Rights upheld the complaint. They found that treatment contrary to his mother's wishes breached his right to physical integrity under article 8 as the hospital had failed to seek the High Court's approval for the proposed treatment.

Permissive declarations

When the court's approval for a plan of care is sought, the method used to authorise treatment is by way of a declaration in which the court declares that the proposed treatment is lawful. A declaration is binding on the parties before the court and doctors and midwives are bound by its terms.

The courts are aware that a declaration may restrict a health professional's ability to exercise their clinical judgement when caring for a baby because, if a court declares that a baby should have no antibiotic therapy, for example, it would be unlawful for the doctor or midwife to give antibiotics.

To avoid such a situation the court resorts to the use of a permissive declaration. This involves the court authorising the withholding of certain treatment at the discretion of the team caring for the baby. It allows treatment to be given where this is in the best interests of the baby, but also allows treatment, even life-sustaining treatment, to be withheld where it is not considered in the baby's best interests.

CASE STUDY: The permissive declaration

In *Re Wyatt (A Child) (Medical Treatment: Continuation of Order)* [2005], the intervention of the court was sought in respect of the medical treatment of a child whose condition had significantly deteriorated; she had developed an intermittent rasping cough and it was likely that she was suffering from a viral infection. Medical experts were of the opinion that the only intervention, if she continued to deteriorate, would be intubation and ventilation, but that it would not be in her best interests as essentially it would be futile. The view of the parents was that, if she were ventilated, she would recover.

The court made it clear that, in the best interests of the child, the care team should be able to refrain from having to intervene by way of intubation and ventilation. The authority was granted by way of a permissive, not mandatory, declaration so that, at the moment the decision arose, the medical authorities were required to use their best judgement in the child's best interests as to whether to withhold the treatment or not. Accordingly, a decision to desist would be lawful.

As a registered midwife, your care and treatment of an infant will be facilitated through the cooperation and consent of a person with parental responsibility and this will usually be a parent of the child. It is essential, therefore, that you are familiar with the rules on parental responsibility and the limits to a person's right to act on behalf of an infant.

The Gillick competent child

The matter of whether a child under 16 has the necessary competence to consent to examination and treatment was decided by the House of Lords in *Gillick v West Norfolk and Wisbech AHA* [1986]. In this case, a mother objected to Department of Health advice that health professionals could give contraceptive advice and treatment to children under 16 without parental consent. The court held that a child under 16 had the ability to consent to medical examination and treatment, including contraceptive treatment, if he or she had sufficient maturity and intelligence to understand the nature and implications of that treatment. The decision on whether a child is competent to give consent is for the midwife providing care and treatment to decide.

The test for Gillick competence

Activity 6.3   *Reflection*

Before reading the next part, make a list of the factors you think should be taken into account when deciding whether a child has sufficient maturity and intelligence to make a healthcare decision.

Please do not move on to the next part until you are ready for the answer.

In determining whether a child has sufficient maturity and intelligence to consent to treatment decisions, midwives need to take account of:

- the child's chronological, emotional and mental age;
- the child's intellectual development;
- the child's ability to reach a decision.

The aim of the Gillick principle is to reflect the transition of a child towards adulthood. The legal competence to make decisions is conditional on the child's gradually acquiring maturity. A relatively young child would have sufficient maturity and intelligence to be capable of consenting to a plaster on a small cut. Equally, a child who had the capacity to consent to dental treatment or the repair of broken bones may lack competence to consent to more serious or complex treatment (*Re R (A Minor) (Wardship Consent to Treatment)* [1992]). To date, no court has ever found that a child has had the competence to refuse life-sustaining treatment (*Re L (Medical Treatment: Gillick Competence)* [1998]).

> ### CASE STUDY: Gillick competence
>
> In *JSC and CHC v Wren* [1987], a pregnant 15-year-old girl obtained approval for a therapeutic abortion. Her parents sought to prevent this by applying to a court for an injunction.
>
> An injunction was refused by the court because the expectant mother in this case had sufficient intelligence and understanding, both of the nature of the proposed treatment and of her obligation to her parents, to make up her own mind. She was Gillick competent.

On the specific issue of contraceptive advice and treatment in *Gillick*, Lord Scarman gave an indication of how midwives should approach the assessment of competence. He said there was much to be understood by a child if they were to have the competence to consent. The midwife giving the advice or treatment would need to be satisfied that not only was the advice understood, but that the child had sufficient maturity to understand what was involved. This would include:

- moral and family questions such as the future relationship with the parents;
- longer-term problems associated with the emotion of pregnancy or its termination;
- the health risks associated with sexual intercourse at a young age.

Where you are satisfied that the child is Gillick competent, the consent of the child is as effective as that of an adult and cannot be overruled by a parent.

Fraser guidelines

Giving contraceptive advice and treatment to a child under 16 years of age gives rise to a concern that a midwife may be accused of procuring sexual intercourse with a child under 16, a criminal offence (Sexual Offences Act 2003). To protect you from such accusations, Lord Fraser in *Gillick* issued guidance to ensure that contraceptive advice and treatment were only given on clinical grounds. There might be exceptional cases when, in the interests of the child's welfare, a midwife might give contraceptive advice and treatment without the permission or even knowledge of the parents. You must be satisfied:

- that the girl understood your advice;
- that you could not persuade her to tell or allow you to tell her parents;
- that she was likely to have sexual intercourse with or without contraceptive treatment;
- that unless she received such advice or treatment her physical or mental health was likely to suffer;
- that her best interests required such advice or treatment without the knowledge or consent of her parents.

It is essential that this guidance is followed in practice to avoid any possibility of criminal conduct.

The defence offered by Lord Fraser's guidance has been extended by the Sexual Offences Act 2003, section 13. This provides a defence against aiding, abetting or counselling a sexual offence if the purpose is to:

- protect the child from sexually transmitted infection;
- protect the physical safety of the child;
- protect the child from becoming pregnant;
- promote the child's emotional well-being by the giving of advice, unless the purpose is to obtain sexual gratification or to cause or encourage the relevant sexual act.

CASE STUDY: Fraser guidelines

In *R (Axon) v Secretary of State for Health* [2006], the court held that there was no reason why the rule in *Gillick* should not apply to other treatment and advice.

The approach of a health professional to a young person seeking advice and treatment on sexual issues without notifying his or her parents should be in accordance with Lord Fraser's guidelines. There was no infringement of the rights of a young person's parents if a health professional was permitted to withhold information relating to the advice or treatment of the young person on sexual matters.

There has been a growing trend in recent years to interchange the terms 'Gillick competent' and 'Fraser competent' as if they were one and the same. This is not the case. The test for Gillick competence provides you with an objective test of competence, as it identifies children under 16 who have the competence to consent to examination and treatment if they demonstrate sufficient maturity and intelligence to understand and appraise the nature and implications of the treatment.

Lord Fraser's guidance only relates to contraception and includes the necessity to ensure that the girl understands the contraceptive advice. However, it otherwise concentrates on the desirability of parental involvement and the enhanced risks of unprotected sex.

Were Gillick completely subsumed into Fraser, the detailed assessment of a child's competence would be lost. Were Fraser subsumed into Gillick, the particular problem of contraception would be lost in the generalities of a child's competence (Wheeler, 2006).

Children 16 or 17 years old

Where midwives have care for a young woman who has attained the age of 16 years, the provisions for consent to treatment are decided by the Family Law Reform Act 1969, section 8.

(1) The consent of a minor who has attained the age of sixteen years to any surgical, medical or dental treatment which, in the absence of consent, would constitute a trespass to his [sic] person, shall be as effective as it would be if he were of full age; and where a minor has by virtue of this section given an effective consent to any treatment it shall not be necessary to obtain any consent for it from his parent or guardian.

(2) In this section 'surgical, medical or dental treatment' includes any procedure undertaken for the purposes of diagnosis, and this section applies to any procedure (including, in particular, the administration of an anaesthetic) which is ancillary to any treatment as it applies to that treatment.

This allows a child of 16 or 17 to give consent as if they were of full age, that is, an adult. Where such consent is given it is as effective as that of an adult. It cannot be overruled by the parent or guardian.

The courts have adopted a very narrow construction of the provisions of section 8 of the 1969 Act. A child to whom the provisions apply can only consent to treatment or examinations that are therapeutic or diagnostic (*Re W (A Minor) (Medical Treatment: Court's Jurisdiction)* [1992]). It does not allow consent for the donation of organs or blood. Even the giving of blood samples is excluded (separate provision is made for these under section 21(2) of the Family Law Reform Act 1969).

Contraceptive advice and treatment and maternity care are considered a legitimate and beneficial treatment under section 5 of the National Health Service Act 1977 and section 41 of the National Health Service (Scotland) Act 1978. A young woman who has attained 16 years can consent to her antenatal, perinatal and postnatal care, contraceptive advice and treatment under this provision.

The assessment of the capacity of a 16- or 17-year-old child to consent to treatment would be in accordance with the provisions of the Mental Capacity Act 2005 and its code of practice (see Chapter 5).

Activity 6.4   Group work

You will have seen that a competent child under 18 years can make treatment decisions and consent to treatment even though the person with parental responsibility objects. Imagine that the same competent child decides to refuse to consent to treatment.

- Discuss in a group the rights of the competent child to refuse treatment and what action can be taken when such a refusal happens.
- During the discussion, please make some notes of the issues raised.

Now read on for further information.

Parents and consent

Although both the courts and Parliament allow children to make treatment decisions for themselves as they mature, no minor (child under 18 years) is wholly autonomous (*Re M (A Child) (Refusal of Medical Treatment)* [1999]). If a child under 18 refuses medical examination or treatment, the law will allow others to consent even if the child is competent.

Lord Donaldson summed up the position thus:

I now prefer the analogy of the legal 'flak jacket' which protects you from claims by the litigious whether you acquire it from your patient, who may be a minor over the age of 16 or a Gillick competent child under that age, or from another person having parental responsibilities which include a right to consent to treatment of the minor.

Anyone who gives you a flak jacket (i.e. consent) may take it back, but then you only need one and so long as you continue to have one you have the legal right to proceed.

(*Re W (A Minor) (Medical Treatment: Court's Jurisdiction)*
[1992], (Lord Donaldson MR at 641)

Where a competent child consents to medical examination or treatment, it cannot be overruled by a parent. However, where the same child refuses to consent, you may obtain consent from another person with parental responsibility who has the right to consent to treatment on the child's behalf, or ultimately from a court.

Restricting a child's liberty

There may be occasions where a child refuses to remain in hospital for the care and treatment they require and the midwife believes there would be a risk of harm if the child were to leave the hospital. Under these circumstances it may be necessary for the midwife to consider the use of the Children Act 1989, section 25, which allows for the use of secure accommodation to restrict the liberty of a child.

Secure accommodation is not defined by the Children Act 1989. It depends on what use is made of the environment rather than having a pre-designated secure area. For example, locking the entrance to a maternity unit, standing in a doorway or preventing a child leaving a room would be using accommodation in a secure way (*Re B (A Minor) (Treatment and Secure Accommodation)* [1997]). The provisions of the Children Act 1989, section 25, apply to local authority homes, residential and nursing homes, and health and educational premises. It allows restriction without a court order for 72 hours in any 28-day period. A record must be kept of the nature and duration of the restriction. Where the period of restriction is going to be longer, a court order is required.

Conditions

Before restricting the liberty of a child you must be satisfied that the child is 13 or older and that the following conditions apply.

- The child has a history of absconding and is likely to abscond from any other description of accommodation.
- If the child absconds, he or she is likely to suffer significant harm.
- If the child is kept in any other description of accommodation, he or she is likely to injure themselves or other persons.

CASE STUDY: *Restricting the liberty of a child*

In *B (A Minor) (Treatment and Secure Accommodation)* [1997], a pregnant 17 year old suffered from a cocaine/crack addiction. She developed pre-eclampsia, which was potentially fatal for her and her unborn child. She also had a phobia about needles, doctors and any medical treatment and wished to discharge herself from hospital. The hospital applied to the court for an order restricting her liberty by locking the door to the maternity unit.

The court allowed the restriction of liberty and held that B's right to refuse to give consent to treatment could be overridden by the court or a person with parental responsibility for her.

The local authority and her mother, having parental responsibility, could take steps to protect her best interests, which could permit the use of reasonable force in order to administer the correct treatment.

The restriction of liberty was the essential factor in determining whether accommodation could be secure accommodation within the meaning of section 25 of the Children Act 1989, so that secure accommodation did not need to be previously designated, but each case would depend on its facts.

- Consent is a state of mind where a person agrees to the touching of their body as part of an examination or treatment.
- Children pass through three developmental stages to becoming an autonomous adult: the infant and child of tender years, the Gillick competent child, and the 16- or 17-year-old child.
- The courts acknowledge that no child under 18 is wholly autonomous. However, the law recognises the right of children to consent to medical treatment as they develop and mature with age.
- A person with parental responsibility is generally entitled to consent to treatment on behalf of an infant and child. There is a small group of important decisions that should not be carried out or arranged by one parent alone.
- Parents' rights must be exercised in the child's best interests. Where those with parental responsibility strongly oppose the giving or withholding of treatment by a health professional to their infant, the matter will need to be referred to the court for a decision. The court may use a permissive declaration to authorise withholding of treatment at the discretion of the team caring for the infant.
- An expectant mother under 16 has the legal competence to consent to examination and treatment if she has sufficient maturity and intelligence to understand the nature and implications of that treatment.
- A young woman who has attained the age of 16 has the right to consent to examination and treatment under the Family Law Reform Act 1969, section 8.
- If a child under 18 refuses medical examination or treatment, the law allows others to consent even if he or she has competence.
- Where a competent child consents to medical examination or treatment, this cannot be overruled by a parent.
- There may be occasions where a child who is pregnant refuses to remain in hospital for treatment. The Children Act 1989, section 25, can be used to restrict liberty if the conditions set out in the section are met.

Knowledge review

Having completed the chapter, how would you now rate your knowledge of the following topics?

	Good	Adequate	Poor
1. The three developmental stages a child passes through to become an autonomous adult.			
2. How the law bestows parental responsibility.			
3. The extent of a person with parental responsibility's right to consent to treatment.			
4. The test for Gillick competence.			

	Good	Adequate	Poor
5. The requirements for a valid consent from a child who is 16 or 17 years old.			

Where you're not confident in your knowledge of a topic, what will you do next?

Further reading

The following is a useful booklet on a wide range of consent issues with children and it can be downloaded from **www.gmc-uk.org/guidance/ethical_guidance/children_ guidance_index.asp**:

General Medical Council (GMC) (2007) *0–18 Years: Guidance for all doctors.* London: GMC.

These two explanatory booklets are designed to help children and parents understand their rights in making decisions about treatment:

Department of Health (DH) (2001) *Consent: A guide for children and young people.* London: DH.

Department of Health (DH) (2001) *Consent: What you have a right to expect: a guide for parents.* London: DH.

To help you meet the legal requirements for consent and children, we recommend this booklet:

Department of Health (DH) (2001) *Seeking Consent: Working with children.* London: DH.

The DH has also produced this booklet about provision of maternity services for teenagers:

Department of Health (DH)/Department of Children, Schools and Families (DCSF) (2009) *Getting Maternity Services Right for Pregnant Teenagers and Young Fathers,* 2nd edn. London: DH/DCSF.

Useful websites

www.medicalprotection.org/uk/factsheets/consent-children The Medical Protection Society supports health professionals when they face litigation, and provides a range of advice sheets on the topic of children and consent.

www.scottishlaw.org.uk/journal/mar2001/sclubgilmar01.pdf The Scottish Law website has a very useful explanation of the provisions for consent and children in Scotland.

Chapter 7

Safeguarding children

NMC Standards for Pre-registration Midwifery Education

This chapter will address the following competencies:

Domain: Effective midwifery practice

- Examine and care for babies with specific health or social needs and refer to other professionals or agencies as appropriate.

Domain: Professional and ethical practice

- Work collaboratively with the wider healthcare team and agencies . . . [which] will include those who work in child protection.

Chapter aims

After reading this chapter, you will be able to:

- describe the five principles of the Children Act 1989;
- define significant harm;
- explain how the law seeks to protect children from sexual exploitation;
- understand the role of the midwife in protecting children;
- describe the powers available to safeguard children from abuse.

Introduction

This chapter examines the role of the law in safeguarding children at risk of significant harm. The chapter begins by considering the disturbing nature of child abuse and its many forms. It goes on to discuss the key principles set out in the Children Act 1989 that promote the welfare and safety of children. The chapter then considers the legal arrangements in place when things go wrong and when children need protection from significant harm.

The United Nations Convention on the Rights of the Child (UN, 1989) requires the government to have regard to the full spectrum of human rights for all children and to consider children in legislative and policy decisions. The Convention defines a child as a person under the age of 18 years. People under 18 are often referred to in law as minors.

Article 19 of the Convention says that children have the right to be protected from abuse and the UK provides this protection through the Children Acts of 1989 and 2004. In spite of a wide range of legislative and policy measures, safeguarding children from abuse continues to be one of the most challenging aspects of midwifery practice.

UNICEF (2003) claims that up to 80 per cent of abuse is meted out by biological parents. Midwives are therefore well placed to identify children who may have been abused or who are at risk of abuse. They are also well placed to recognise when parents or other adults have problems that might affect their capacity to fulfil their roles with children safely.

Midwives must know when to refer a child for help as a *child in need* (Children Act 1989, s17) and how to act on concerns that a child is at risk of significant harm through abuse or neglect (Children Act 1989, s31(10)).

Child abuse

An estimated 300 million children worldwide are subjected to violence, exploitation and abuse. In Europe in 2003, UNICEF (2003) reported that two children died from abuse and neglect every week in Germany and the UK, and three a week in France. UK figures for 2008–09 show that there were 41,780 children on child protection registers or subject to child protection plans because they were at risk of abuse (NSPCC, 2009). A recent review by the Care Quality Commission (CQC) in England reported that, of the 34,000 children needing protection in 2007–08, 45 per cent were as a result of neglect, 15 per cent as a result of physical abuse and 25 per cent as a result of emotional abuse (CQC, 2009).

The child protection register is a list of children who are at risk of abuse. The register acts as an alert that these children need a child protection plan to keep them safe from abuse. Each child whose name is on the register will have a plan agreed by parents and social workers to help keep them safe. The plan states the intended outcomes for the child and what individuals involved in the case, including parents, will do to make the plan work.

The categories of abuse listed on the register are:

- **neglect** – the persistent failure to meet a child's basic physical and/or psychological needs, which is likely to result in the serious impairment of the child's health or development;
- **physical abuse** – involves hitting, shaking, throwing, poisoning, burning, scalding, drowning, suffocating or causing other physical harm to a child (this includes Munchhausen syndrome by proxy);
- **sexual abuse** – involves forcing or enticing a child or young person to take part in sexual activities, whether they involve physical contact or not;
- **emotional abuse** – persistent emotional ill-treatment of a child such as to cause severe and persistent adverse effects on the child's emotional development.

CASE STUDY: Categories of child abuse

Neglect

The parents of five children were jailed for seven years after admitting child cruelty. The couple left their children – one-year-old twins, a three year old, a four year old and a seven year old – in excrement-smeared bedrooms while they apparently lived in comfort surrounded by modern electronic products. The children's plight came to light when an ambulance was called when one of the twins appeared lifeless (reported in *The Telegraph*, 24 November 2004).

Physical abuse

Seventeen-month-old Baby P suffered horrific and systematic abuse at the hands of his mother, lover and lodger before his death, in spite of being monitored by social workers. All three were found guilty and jailed for the death of Baby P (*R v B* [2010]).

Sexual abuse

In *R v B* [2001], a man was sentenced to nine months' imprisonment for taking indecent photographs of a child.

A nursery worker was jailed for seven years as part of an indeterminate sentence for the sexual abuse of young children in her care at the nursery.

Emotional abuse

In *Re B (Children) (Emotional Welfare: Interim Care Order)* [2002], the Court of Appeal upheld an interim care order on two children on the grounds of emotional abuse, because their father had made persistent threats to their lives during an acrimonious period of separation from their mother.

The category of concern is important. Midwives must identify evidence of a risk of significant harm before a child's name is placed on a register. In *R v Hampshire County Council* [1999], the Court of Appeal held that, before a child was placed on the child protection register, there had to be evidence of significant harm, or a risk of such harm, in relation to the category of abuse under which the child was to be registered. For emotional abuse, midwives would have to be satisfied, on the evidence before them, that a child was at risk of suffering persistent or severe emotional ill-treatment or rejection.

It is not enough to identify a stressful family situation: there must be evidence of risk of significant harm to the child.

The Children Act 1989

The aim of the Children Act 1989 was to provide an effective legal framework for the safety and protection of children. It enshrines five main principles:

- the welfare principle;
- keeping the family together;
- the non-intervention principle;
- unified laws and procedures;
- avoidance of delay.

The welfare principle

The welfare principle states that, when a court determines any question with regard to the upbringing of a child or its property, the child's welfare shall be the court's paramount consideration (Children Act 1989, s1).

Activity 7.3   *Reflection*

'Welfare' and 'paramount' are two terms that stand out in the courts' duty to children under the Children Act 1989.

- Note down what you consider the terms 'paramount' and 'welfare' to mean.

Please do not move on to the next part until you are ready for the answer.

'Paramount' means more than the child being the first of a list of considerations by the court. In *J v C* [1970], the court held that 'paramount' means:

> [m]ore than placing the child's welfare first. It connotes a process where the course to be followed will be that which is most in the interests of the child's welfare.

It is the only consideration of the court and the duty to consider the welfare of the child will be reflected in the court's decision.

Welfare is not statutorily defined by the Children Act 1989 and the court is able to exercise its discretion in each case. It is not uncommon for the court to speak of acting in the best interests of the child. The Court of Appeal will only overrule a decision on the welfare principle where it considers it to be plainly wrong (*G V G (Minors) (Custody Appeal)* [1985]).

CASE STUDY: Welfare principle

In Re W (A Minor) (Residence Order) [1992], a couple agreed before their child was born that she would live with her father. Two days after the birth a parental responsibility agreement gave the father parental rights, but the mother then changed her mind and applied for the return of the child.

    When the judge declined to move the baby pending a report and final determination of the case, the mother appealed. The Court of Appeal held that, although there was no presumption that any child of any age was better off with one parent than the other, it was a rebuttable fact that a tiny baby's interests were best served by being with its mother. The judge was plainly wrong to leave the question of the child's placement until the final hearing, as the child was less than a month old and her welfare required that she should be with her mother.

In child proceedings the court must consider a checklist of factors to help it determine what would be in the best interests of the child's welfare (Children Act 1989, s1(4)). The checklist encourages the court to consider all factors in a holistic way and can help people with a child protection role, such as midwives, to focus on the relevant issues.

Activity 7.4   *Critical thinking*

You have already written what the term 'welfare' means. Imagine that you have been asked to decide on the best interests of a child's welfare.

- In a group or individually discuss what factors you would take into account in making such a decision. For example, will you allow the child to express his or her wishes?

Please do not move on to the next part until you are ready for the answer.

The welfare checklist requires the court to have regard to the following.

- **The ascertainable wishes and feelings of the child.**
  These will be considered in the light of the child's age and understanding (*Gillick v West Norfolk and Wisbech AHA* [1986]; see Chapter 6). Unless the child can show sufficient maturity and understanding to exercise a wise choice on the issues, the court will appoint a Children's Guardian, an independent officer of the Children and Family Court Advisory and Support Service experienced in working with children and families, to represent the interests of the child (*Re S (A Minor) (Representation)* [1993]).

- **The child's physical, emotional and educational needs.**
  The court is required to take a wide-ranging view of the needs of the child that go beyond material and monetary needs. As Lord Justice Griffiths (at 637) stated in *Re P (Adoption: Parental Agreement)* [1985], *Anyone with experience of life knows that affluence and happiness are not necessarily synonymous.*

- **The likely effect of any change in circumstances.**
  The court must consider the impact of change on the child and is encouraged to avoid unnecessary disruption to the life of the child. In *Re B (Minors) (Residence*

Order) [1992], the mother of four children left the family home, leaving them with their father. She later returned and removed one of the children. The Court of Appeal held that an order for the return of a child to his father and siblings could be made in order to minimise the effect of a change of circumstances on the child.

- **The age, sex, background and any characteristics of the child that the court considers relevant.**
  The age and sex of the child will not conclusively determine the welfare of the child but can be influential. In *Re S (A Minor) (Custody)* [1991], a mother was granted custody of a child even though she had previously assaulted the child and had then disappeared for several weeks leaving the very young child with its father. The Court of Appeal held that there was no presumption that one parent was to be preferred over the other for the purposes of looking after a child. Although it might be expected that young children, especially girls, would remain with their mothers, where there was a dispute over custody this was merely a consideration rather than a presumption.

- **The harm suffered or that the child is at risk of suffering.**
  In *Re G (Children) (Same Sex Partner)* [2006], the court refused to allow a woman and her two children to relocate from the Midlands to Cornwall when her relationship with her same-sex partner broke down. The court held that, in the case of a same-sex relationship where the care of the children was shared, the children would not distinguish between one woman and another on the grounds of a biological relationship. Therefore, it was necessary for the court in making its determination on the welfare of the children to balance the harm to the children of not allowing the move against the future harm to the children if they were not able to have the relationship with the estranged partner that they needed for their welfare.

- **How capable each parent, and any other person, is of meeting the child's needs.**
  In *Humberside County Council v B* [1993], the Court of Appeal held that a court had been wrong to issue an interim care order against the parents, who both suffered from schizophrenia. The Court concluded that the magistrates had failed to consider the capability of the parents when determining the welfare of the child.

- **The range of powers available to the court under this Act.**
  This provision requires the court to consider how best to provide for the child's welfare. It is not confined to considering the order requested by the local authority and can instead substitute a different order or no order at all. In *Re O (A Child) (Supervision Order: Future Harm)* [2001], the court substituted a supervision order in place of the care order sought by the local authority as, on the evidence, what was required to protect the child was support and a watching brief on the family, where the mother suffered from recurring episodes of mental health problems that might result in future risk of harm to the child.

Courts must clearly demonstrate that they have considered each element of the welfare checklist when making a decision about the welfare of the child.

Keeping the family together

The Children Act 1989 has a presumption that a child is best looked after within a family where both parents play an equal part. Where difficulties occur, families should be supported to carry out that role unless it is clearly against the best interests of the child. Before the introduction of the Act, social services departments were seen as needlessly adversarial, with removal of children from the family being the main solution to problems within the family.

Now a range of family support mechanisms and the involvement of other family members are used to provide a nurturing and protective environment for children. In the first five years of the Children Act 1989 there were 20,000 fewer children in the care system.

Local authorities have a duty to promote the welfare of a child in need by providing appropriate services (Children Act 1989, s17). The aim is to promote the upbringing of such children by their families.

Activity 7.5   Group work

In a group discuss what you consider the meaning of a child in need to be. Write down key points that will indicate that a child is in need.

Please do not read the text below until you have completed this activity.

A child in need is one who:

[i]s unlikely to achieve or maintain a reasonable standard of health or develop-ment without the provision of services by a local authority or their health or development is likely to be significantly impaired or further impaired without the provision of services by a local authority or they are disabled.

(Children Act 1989, s17(10))

The definition includes not only children at risk of abuse, but also other children. For example, a child who is disabled may meet the definition of a child in need but is not necessarily at risk of abuse. The duty to children in need is key to preventative work with particularly vulnerable children. Midwives are ideally placed to help identify children who would benefit from intervention by the local authority. Good practice requires the local authority to assess need in an open way that involves the child and their carers. Families have a right to receive sympathetic support and sensitive intervention in their life (DH, 1997a).

The non-intervention principle

The Children Act 1989, section 1(5), provides that a court shall not make an order unless it considers that doing so would be better for the child than making no order at all. The non-intervention or no order principle is one of the most innovative principles of the Act (Bainham, 1990). It requires the court to be satisfied that any order it issues will make a positive contribution to the welfare of the child. This helps avoid unnecessary state intervention and preserves the integrity and independence of the family. As Justice Wall stated in *Re DH (A Minor) (Child Abuse)* [1994] at p707:

Parents should be free wherever possible to bring up their children without interference from courts or other statutory body.

Where midwives are involved in child protection proceedings, they must take note of the non-intervention principle and the initial presumption of the court that no order will be issued. It will be for the agencies involved to rebut this presumption by demonstrating that the grounds for an order are met and that the order is necessary to promote the welfare of the child.

Unified laws and procedures

The Children Act 1989 unifies the laws and procedures relating to the welfare of children. Previously there existed distinct private and public law systems. Now there is one set of laws that includes provision for both private law matters, where there are disputes within families that cannot be resolved without recourse to the law, and public law provision that allows for the protection of children suffering significant harm.

The aim of the five principles of the Children Act 1989 is to ensure that matters of concern regarding children are managed sensitively and with appropriate speed for the benefit of the welfare of the child. This ensures that the child is viewed by the law and practitioners as a person, not an object of concern (Butler-Sloss, 2003).

Avoidance of delay

Delays in child care cases are considered detrimental to the child concerned. Children require stability and prolonged litigation is damaging. Under the Children Act 1989, courts may be accessed according to the degree of complexity of the case. In applications for care and supervision orders, courts are required to draw up a timetable for disposal of the case. There is a presumption that a full hearing will take place in 12 weeks. The Court of Appeal held in *B v B (Minors) (Residence and Care Disputes)* [1994] that practitioners had a duty to avoid delay in child cases. Where midwives are asked to provide reports or statements as proof of evidence, they must do so without delay.

The Act introduced a three-tier court system where cases could be moved according to complexity in order to avoid delay.

Magistrates' courts

Children Act cases are heard by a family proceedings court. The bench is drawn from magistrates on the criminal bench and the youth court. All applications for care or supervision orders under the Children Act 1989 start in the family proceedings court.

County courts

These courts deal with a wide variety of civil cases, including family proceedings. Cases are normally heard by a judge. Around 50 county courts are designated care centres where specially nominated care judges hear care order applications transferred from the magistrates' courts. A number of county courts are family hearing centres, which deal with contested private law hearings, such as with whom a child should live, and adoption applications. Divorce county courts are able to hear applications relating to children arising out of divorce proceedings.

Any county court may make orders under the Children Act 1989 in the course of other family proceedings, such as when orders need to be made regarding children following an application by a parent for a non-molestation order under the Family Law Act 1996.

The High Court's civil jurisdiction

The Family Division of the High Court hears family proceedings, including Children Act and adoption cases, and appeals from family proceedings courts. Where urgent cases need to be considered, the Court operates an out of court hours service and there is always a High Court judge on-call.

Significant harm

Activity 7.6	Group work

In a group discuss what factors you would take into account when determining if a child is suffering or is likely to suffer significant harm. Remember to look at factors that may cause significant harm now and factors that could cause significant harm in the future. Separate your list into present harm and future harm. Some factors may be present in both lists.

Please do not read the text below until you have completed this activity.

Prior to the Children Act 1989, there were 17 routes into care. The welfare principle alone is not robust enough to act as the threshold for state intervention in family life. There must at least be a risk of significant harm to the child before state intervention in a family's life is justified.

Significant harm is not defined in the Children Act 1989. When the proposed bill was debated in the House of Lords, the Lord Chancellor said:

> It speaks of significant harm – namely that which, being more than minimal, indicates that compulsory care or supervision may be justified.

Significant harm describes the threshold criteria below which state intervention with families cannot be justified. Two requirements are necessary:

- the child is suffering or is likely to suffer significant harm (Children Act 1989, s31(2));
- the harm is attributable to a lack of reasonable parental care.

The phrase is expressed in the present and the future tense. The present tense refers to harm suffered at the time immediately preceding intervention by the child protection authorities.

CASE STUDY: Applying the threshold criteria

In *Re M (A Minor) (Care Order: Threshold Conditions)* [1994], a court held that the significant harm criteria no longer applied after a father killed the mother of a baby who was now being looked after by an aunt. The father was serving life in prison and was therefore no longer a risk to the baby.

The future tense element of the threshold criteria relies on speculation about the likelihood of harm. That is, there must be a real possibility of harm to the child. It need not be proved that the child is more likely to be harmed than not. The standard of proof is the normal civil standard based on the balance of probabilities, not the criminal standard requiring evidence beyond reasonable doubt (*Re H (Minors) (Sexual Abuse: Standard of Proof)* [1996]). However, the House of Lords states that the more serious the allegation the less likely it is to have happened and the more sceptical the courts should be. More evidence is required by the courts to prove more serious allegations.

It is not necessary to establish who caused harm to the child. If the harm is attributable to a third party, it will only be actionable in care or supervision proceedings if it could reasonably have been prevented by the parent.

To satisfy the threshold criteria for state intervention the harm must be significant. This definition incorporates physical and emotional harm and neglect. For example, in *Re O (A Minor) (Care Order: Education Procedure)* [1992], the court held that truanting amounted to harm that could be significant. Minor shortcomings in healthcare or minor deficits in physical, psychological or social development should not require compulsory intervention unless cumulatively they are having, or are likely to have, serious and lasting effects upon the child (DH, 1997a). Where the harm relates to health or development, the child is compared with a similar child (Children Act 1989, s31(10)). The need to use a standard appropriate to the child in question arises because some children have characteristics or developmental difficulties that mean that they cannot be expected to be as healthy or well developed as others.

To meet the threshold criteria, the Children Act 1989 requires that the significant harm is attributable either to unreasonable care or to the child being beyond parental control.

Care refers to the physical and emotional support that a reasonable parent would give to the particular child having regard to their needs (*Re B (A Minor) (Care Order: Criteria)* [1993]). Where the child is beyond parental control, the fault or innocence of the parents is irrelevant (*Re O (A Minor) (Care Order: Education Procedure)* [1992]).

Sexual offences against children

Of all crimes, sexual crimes are the ones that are generally viewed with revulsion because of their intimate nature and enduring effect on the victims. This revulsion is particularly heightened when sexual offences are committed against children.

To strengthen and modernise the law relating to sexual activity, Parliament introduced the Sexual Offences Act 2003, which seeks to extend protection from sexual exploitation for children and vulnerable adults. Child and vulnerable adult protection is now an integral part of a midwife's role, so it is essential that you are aware of the key provisions of the 2003 Act in order to recognise and support victims of unlawful sexual activity.

Activity 7.7   *Reflection and research*

- Before reading on, make a list of activities you would consider to be sexual activities. (For example, if you consider kissing to be a sexual activity you should add it to your list.)
- When you are satisfied with your list, compare it to the legal definition of sexual activity given in the Sexual Offences Act 2003 below.

Please do not read the text below until you have completed this activity.

Sexual activity

According to the Sexual Offences Act 2003, an activity is sexual if a reasonable person considers that:

[w]hatever the circumstances or a person's purpose the act is because of its nature sexual. This would include activities such as sexual intercourse, kissing, masturbation and intimate touching as they are by their very nature sexual.

Offences against children

The preamble to the Sexual Offences Act 2003 states that its purpose is to *make provision about sexual offences, their prevention and the protection of children from other sexual acts.* The Act creates specific offences against children in three age categories and makes the issue of consent irrelevant in each case – that is, the offence is committed regardless of whether or not the child consents.

CASE STUDY: An offence is committed regardless of the child's consent

In *R v A* [2005], a 15-year-old boy was sentenced to seven years' detention for raping a child under 13. The boy had met his victim, who was 11, through an internet chatroom. Over a period of two days he had sexual intercourse with the girl on four occasions, once in a cinema, once at her home and twice in the changing rooms of clothes shops. He believed that the girl had been a willing participant in the sexual activity that had taken place. Her willingness was, however, irrelevant due to her age, and she was easily impressionable.

Protecting children under 13

Children under 13 are now regarded in law as being incapable of consenting to any form of sexual activity under any circumstances. Therefore, provisions to protect children under 13 apply the main non-consensual sexual offences to those who engage in sexual activity with a child who is 12 or under.

Concept summary: Offences against children under 13

Sections 5–8 of the Sexual Offences Act 2003 state the following.

- **Rape of a child under 13**
  It is an offence for a person intentionally to penetrate with his penis the vagina, anus or mouth of a child under 13.

- **Assault of a child under 13 by penetration**
  It is an offence for a person intentionally to penetrate sexually the vagina or anus of a child under 13 with a part of his body, or with anything else.

- **Sexual assault of a child under 13**
  It is an offence for a person to touch sexually a child under 13.

- **Causing or inciting a child under 13 to engage in sexual activity**
  It is an offence for a person intentionally to cause or incite a child under the age of 13 to engage in sexual activity.

These offences are strictly related to age and the prosecution only has to prove that the sexual activity took place and that the child was under 13 at the time of the offence. It is not a defence to claim that they had a reasonable, if mistaken, belief that the child was over 13.

When sexual activity involves a child under 13, consent is not an issue and is irrelevant to the charge, but it can be taken into account by the judge when passing sentence. It is open to the prosecutors to exercise discretion where the defendant is a child. The overriding public concern is to protect children, and it was not Parliament's intention to punish children unnecessarily or for the criminal law to intervene where it is wholly inappropriate.

Under the Criminal Justice Act 2003 only Crown Prosecutors may decide whether a person under 18 can be charged with a sexual offence under the Sexual Offences Act 2003. In any case, where there is sufficient evidence of a sexual offence committed by a child to justify instituting proceedings, the public interest must be considered with care before any prosecution is commenced.

Prosecutors must have as much information as possible from sources such as the police, youth offending teams and any professionals, including health professionals, assisting those agencies about the defendant's home circumstances and the circumstances surrounding the alleged offence, as well as any information known about the victim (*R v Chief Constable of Kent ex parte L* [1991]).

Such factors as the age and understanding of the offender, the relevant ages of the parties, whether the complainant entered into sexual activity willingly, the relationship between the parties and its nature and duration, and whether this represents a genuine transitory phase of adolescent development, and what is in the best interests and welfare of the children involved will be considered before a decision on prosecution is made.

Protecting children under 16

The age of consent is now 16 years. Offences that specifically aim to protect children under this age state that sexual activity even with consent is unlawful.

Concept summary: Offences against children under 16

Sections 9–12 of the Sexual Offences Act 2003 state the following.

- **Sexual activity with a child**
  It is an offence for a person aged 18 or over to intentionally touch a child under 16, the touching is sexual, and the defendant does not reasonably believe that the child is 16 or over.

- **Causing or inciting a child to engage in sexual activity**
  It is an offence for a person aged 18 or over to intentionally cause or incite another a child under 16 to engage in an activity, the activity is sexual, and the defendant does not reasonably believe that the child is 16 or over.

- **Engaging in sexual activity in the presence of a child**
  It is an offence for a person aged 18 or over to intentionally engage in sexual activity to obtain sexual gratification when a child under 16 is present or can observe. The defendant knows or believes that the child is aware of the activity or intends that they should be aware and the defendant does not reasonably believe that the child is 16 or over.

- **Causing a child to watch a sexual act**
  It is an offence for a person aged 18 or over to intentionally cause a child under 16 to watch another person engaging in an activity, or to look at an image of any person engaging in an activity for the defendant's sexual gratification and the defendant does not reasonably believe that the child is 16 or over.

Although the main provisions are aimed at protecting children under 16 from exploitation by adults, the offences can be committed by children under 18 but are subject to a reduced penalty (Sexual Offences Act 2003, s13). However, Crown Prosecution Service guidance states that the provisions are designed to protect children, not punish them unnecessarily. Children under 18 will not be prosecuted or issued with a reprimand or final warning where sexual activity was entirely mutually agreed and non-exploitative (CPS, 2004). Prosecutions are possible, however, to protect vulnerable victims.

CASE STUDY: An under-age defendant

In E v DPP [2005], the court held that a boy of 15 had been properly convicted of having unlawful sexual intercourse with a girl of the same age, as girls ran the risk of unwanted pregnancy and so the law needed to deter boys from such activity.

Protecting children under 18

Although the age of consent for sexual activity is generally 16 years, the Sexual Offences Act 2003 seeks to protect children under 18 from sexual exploitation from adults in positions of trust. The Act created a range of offences against children under 18 that would be committed by people in positions of trust. More about the offence of an abuse of position of trust can be found in Chapter 11.

Health and contraceptive advice and treatment for children

Although it has been seen that sexual activity with a child under 16 is unlawful, the Sexual Offences Act 2003 does provide midwives with a defence against aiding, abetting or counselling an offence if the purpose is to:

- protect the child from sexually transmitted infection;
- protect the physical safety of the child;
- protect the child from becoming pregnant;
- promote the child's emotional well-being by the giving of advice, unless the purpose is to obtain sexual gratification or to cause or encourage the relevant sexual act.

Powers to safeguard children

Urgent intervention

The need for timely intervention is crucial to the proper protection of children at risk of significant harm.

CASE STUDY: Failure to act

In Z v United Kingdom [2001], Z and his three siblings had been subjected to severe long-term neglect and abuse. The behaviour of the family had been reported to the social services on several occasions, yet they had only acted five years after the first complaint, when the children were placed in emergency care at the insistence of their mother. The court held that the system had failed to protect Z and his siblings, as the state had clearly failed in its obligation to protect the children from ill-treatment of which it had, or ought to have had, knowledge.

Before you move on to the next part of this chapter, consider what actions can be taken and by whom in the following situations.

- A child is being abused and is in need of urgent intervention.
- A mother walked on to a ward and took her sick child away despite being told that the child was severely ill.

Please do not read the text below until you have completed this activity.

Emergency protection orders

Protection for children in urgent need of intervention is provided by an emergency protection order under the Children Act 1989, section 44. The order is intended for use in an emergency rather than as a routine response to concerns about a child or a measure to coerce parents to cooperate with the local authority.

A court may make the order to any person where it is satisfied that there is reasonable cause to believe that the child is likely to suffer significant harm if they are not removed to accommodation provided by the applicant or if they remain where they are being accommodated. The applicant must convince the court of the urgency of the situation. Proof that a child has suffered significant harm in the past will not satisfy the grounds for the order. Emergency protection must be needed in the current circumstances the child faces, not past dangers.

A court may also grant an emergency protection order where enquiries by the local authority or an authorised person (an officer of the NSPCC) are being unreasonably frustrated and they are unable to establish whether the child is at risk of significant harm.

Effect of an emergency protection order

An emergency protection order operates as a direction to comply with a request to produce the child and can include a provision requiring a person to disclose information about the whereabouts of the child (Children Act 1989, s48). It may authorise the applicant to enter and search for the child named in the order. Should another child be found on the premises, the order will apply to them as well. It is an offence to obstruct the execution of an order.

The emergency protection order authorises the removal of the child or prevents the child's removal from any hospital or other place. It allows the applicant to see the child and, if necessary, remove them from the home. The court may order that a doctor or a registered midwife accompany the applicant. If the child is produced unharmed, with no likelihood of significant harm, they should not be removed.

If the child is removed, parental responsibility is conferred on the applicant for the duration of the order. The order can last for up to eight days and can be renewed for up to a further seven days. Contact by those with parental responsibility cannot be prevented unless specifically directed in the order. There is no right of appeal against the order, but the parents can apply to have it discharged after the initial 72-hour period has elapsed.

As an alternative to removing the child, a court may include an exclusion requirement in an emergency protection order. This allows a perpetrator to be removed from the home instead of the child. To grant the order the court must be satisfied that there is reasonable cause to believe that, if the person is excluded, the child will cease to suffer significant harm or enquiries will cease to be frustrated. There must be another person living in the home who is both able and willing to care for the child.

Police protection

In *X v Liverpool City Council & the Chief Constable of Merseyside Police* [2005], the Court held that the removal of children from their family in an emergency should usually be carried out by means of an emergency protection order as it requires a magistrate to scrutinise the evidence for action before granting an order.

Where an order is not practical, police officers may use their powers under the Children Act 1989, section 46. Where police officers have reasonable cause to believe that a child would be likely to suffer significant harm, they may remove the child to suitable accommodation or prevent the child's removal from any hospital, or other place, in which they are being accommodated. The power allows police officers to take immediate action without the need for a court order. A child made subject to these powers cannot be kept in police protection for more than 72 hours and no parental responsibility is conferred on the police. A constable using the powers must inform the local authority of the steps that have been taken and the reasons for them. If the child is capable of understanding, he or she must also be informed and the officer must take steps to discover the wishes and feelings of the child. As soon as practicable the constable will contact the child's parents and inform them of use of the order and what further steps may be taken with respect to the child. Every police force has an officer designated to inquire further into cases where the police powers have been used.

Duty to investigate

The use of an emergency protection order or police powers begins a process of continued investigation and assessment of the child's welfare. A local authority has a duty to make such enquiries as it considers necessary to enable it to decide whether to take further action to protect a child from harm or promote the welfare of a child (Children Act 1989, s47). This duty arises where the authority is informed that a child in its area is the subject of an emergency protection order or police protection.

The local authority must also investigate where it has reasonable cause to suspect that a child is at risk of significant harm. A local authority must treat as serious allegations of abuse raised with it by nurses, midwives or teachers.

CASE STUDY: Local authority intervention

In *Re E (Children) (Care Proceedings: Social Work Practice)* [2000], a local authority applied for care orders in respect of three children who had been physically ill-treated and showed signs of emotional disturbance. Social services had originally supported the children, but despite warnings from teachers and without proper consideration of the file, had decided to take no further action because of the parents' failure to cooperate. The case had been reopened after another referral from a concerned school and an emergency protection order was made in respect of two of the children and care proceedings were commenced in respect of all the children.

The need to ensure effective interagency working to protect children has now been placed on a statutory footing with the introduction of the Children Act 2004.

Children Act 2004

The aim of the government's strategy for reforming children's services (DH, 2003b) is to ensure that children have the support they need to:

- be healthy;
- stay safe;
- enjoy and achieve through learning;
- make a positive contribution to society;
- achieve economic well-being.

The Children Act 2004 provides the legal framework for this reform and acknowledges that children can only be properly safeguarded if key agencies work together effectively. Local Safeguarding Children Boards (LSCBs) now oversee the way agencies work together to promote the welfare of children (Children Act 2004, s31).

The investigation of allegations of abuse and subsequent intervention with the child and family are now conducted in accordance with the policies and procedures established by the LSCB (HM Government, 2006).

The Children Act 1989 places a duty on health, education and other services to help the local authority to carry out its enquiries under section 47 of the Act. Professionals, including midwives, who participate in these enquiries are assisted in fulfilling their roles by guidance set out in *Working Together to Safeguard Children* (HM Government, 2006).

In the great majority of cases, children remain with their families following an enquiry into an allegation of abuse, even though concerns about abuse or neglect have been substantiated. By encouraging cooperation and respect between agencies and families under investigation, it is hoped that constructive working relationships with families will be developed.

Child assessment orders

A child assessment order may be sought where a child's health, development or treatment is a cause for real concern but who is not regarded by the local authority to be in need of urgent intervention. The order is used where repeated attempts to examine and assess the child have failed. Before granting the order the court must be satisfied there is reasonable cause to suspect that the child is at risk of significant harm and that an assessment to determine this is unlikely to be made without the order (Children Act 1989, s43(1)). When granting the order the court will state the date on which the assessment will commence, and the order will expire seven days from that date. The effect of the order is to require the child to be produced for assessment. A child subject to an assessment order may only be kept away from home if it is necessary for the purposes of the assessment and only for the period specified in the order. The child cannot be kept away from home for the convenience of those operating the assessment.

Once the assessment is completed the local authority will decide how to proceed following discussions with those who have been significantly involved in the enquiries, and this includes the child and its parents. Where it is judged that a child may continue to be at risk of suffering significant harm, a child protection conference will be convened (HM Government, 2006).

The initial child protection conference is responsible for agreeing an outline child protection plan (HM Government, 2006) aimed at:

- ensuring that the child is safe and preventing them from suffering further harm;
- promoting the child's health and development;

- supporting the family and wider family members in safeguarding and promoting the welfare of their child.

Where there is concern that a child continues to suffer, or is at risk of suffering, significant harm, the local authority (or NSPCC) may apply to the court for a care and supervision order (Children Act 1989, s31).

Care or supervision orders

Care or supervision orders are the only route into care, and there is no way to avoid them. The courts cannot use their wardship jurisdiction to compel local authorities to look after children (Children Act 1989, s100). Similarly, a residence order that settles where a child should live cannot be granted in favour of a local authority (Children Act 1989, s9(2)).

A court cannot make a care order on its own motion. It has no power to force a local authority to take a child into care (Re K [1995]).

A court may make a care or supervision order if:

- the child is, or is likely to, suffer significant harm;
- the harm is attributable either to unreasonable care (present or potential) or to the child being beyond parental control.

Once the court has established the threshold criteria have been satisfied, it is able to make a care or supervision order under section 31 of the Children Act 1989 if it is in the best interests of the child's welfare to do so. To reach a decision, the court will scrutinise any plan that the local authority has for the care of the child should the order be granted. This must include plans for continued contact with the child's parents, unless the application for the order specifically requests that all contact should be curtailed (Re T (1994)).

Once the order is made, the court hands over the care of the child to the local authority and it no longer has supervision over the local authority's exercise of the care order (S (Children) (Care Order: Implementation of Care Plan) [2002]).

In care or supervision proceedings the court is being asked to make a long-term order for the protection of the child. The effects of the two orders are different, even though the grounds for granting them are the same. The choice of order depends on the amount of intervention needed to ensure the child's safety.

A supervision order

Under this order a child would be placed under the supervision of the local authority or a probation officer. That person's duty would be to befriend, advise, assist and supervise the child. Parental responsibility is not granted to the local authority and the child cannot be removed from the family home. The court can impose a wide range of health-related requirements in a supervision order that authorise medical examination and assessment and, in some cases, treatment for the child. A supervision order initially runs for a year and may be extended up to a maximum of three years (Children Act 1989, s35(1) and part 1, schedule 3).

A care order

Under a care order a local authority receives a child into its care and takes control of its life. The authority gains parental responsibility for the child and, although parents do not lose their parental responsibility, the local authority can control how they exercise it in relation to their child (Children Act 1989, s33 (2)).

Once the order is made, the local authority controls the care of the child absolutely, free from court scrutiny. The care order will be carried out in accordance with the care plan agreed by the court and, where necessary, this can include removing the child from the family home immediately or at a later date, where a lack of cooperation or continued risk of significant harm makes this necessary. Care orders, which generally cannot be made in respect of a child over 17 or 16 if married, are usually in force until the child is 18 or a court grants an application to have it removed.

Care orders provide for longer-term intervention in a child's life to promote the child's welfare and protect the him or her from significant harm.

The role of the midwife in safeguarding children

There is considerable emphasis on the promotion of the welfare of the child in the guidelines on child protection and safeguarding children and this goes beyond the protection of the child and recognition of abuse. However, it is accepted that dealing with abuse and recognising its signs is not easy. Midwives should consider the need to discuss safeguarding issues as an integral part of practice. It is also advisable that midwives work with those who care for vulnerable mothers. Lazenbatt (2010), in a study conducted in Northern Ireland, concluded that many women may not spontaneously disclose child or domestic abuse and that midwives need to deal with such situations in a supportive, non-coercive and non-judgemental manner.

CHAPTER SUMMARY

- The United Nations Convention on the Rights of the Child requires the government to have regard to the full spectrum of human rights for all children (including the right to be protected from abuse) and to consider children in legislative and policy decisions.
- UK figures indicate that, in 2008–09, there were 41,780 children on child protection registers as being at risk of abuse.
- Midwives have a key role in the identification of children who may have been abused or who are at risk of abuse.
- The Children Act 1989 enshrines the five key principles: holding the child's welfare as paramount, keeping the family together, only intervening where it would make a significant contribution to the welfare of the child, avoiding delay, and unifying laws and procedures.
- The minimum requirement that has to be fulfilled before state intervention in a family's life is the risk of significant harm to the child.
- In reforming children's services, the government aims to ensure that children are able to be healthy, stay safe, enjoy and achieve through learning, make a positive contribution to society and achieve economic well-being.
- Midwives have a role in recognising and preventing the sexual abuse of children. They may also find themselves in the position of providing contraceptive advice and treatment to girls who are under the age of 16. This is lawful if it can be shown to be for the protection of the child concerned.

Knowledge review

Having completed the chapter, how would you now rate your knowledge of the following topics?

	Good	Adequate	Poor
1. The five principles of the Children Act 1989.			
2. The concept of significant harm.			
3. The role of the midwife in protecting children.			
4. The powers available to safeguard children from abuse.			

Where you're not confident in your knowledge of a topic, what will you do next?

Further reading

For a more in-depth review of the application of safeguarding procedures for children we recommend:

Care Quality Commission (CQC) (2009) *Safeguarding Children: A review of arrangements in the NHS for safeguarding children.* London: CQC.

Department of Health (DH) (1997) *Children Act 1989: Guidance and regulations.* London: HMSO.

Department of Health (DH) (2003) *Every Child Matters* (Cm 5860). London: The Stationery Office.

Healthcare Inspectorate Wales (2009) *Safeguarding and Protecting Children in Wales: A review of the arrangements in place across the Welsh National Health Service.* Available online at www.hiw.org.uk.

For those who wish to explore further the effects of childhood abuse on women, we recommend the following:

Bass, E and Davis, L (2002) *The Courage to Heal: A guide for women survivors of child sexual abuse.* London: Vermillion.

Briscoe, C (2009) *Ugly.* London: Hodder.
A heartrending – and ultimately triumphant – story of a child's battle to survive abuse and exploitation.

Useful websites

www.everychildmatters.gov.uk/strategy/guidance Every Child Matters gives a wide range of information and advice on matters relating to safeguarding children in England and Wales.

www.opsi.gov.uk/acts/acts1989/Ukpga_19890041_en_1.htm An online version of the Children Act 1989 from the Office of Public Sector Information.

www.unicef.org/crc UNICEF Convention on the Rights of the Child gives details of the Convention and further information on how its provisions are being promoted throughout the world.

Chapter 8

Record keeping

NMC Standards for Pre-registration Midwifery Education

This chapter will address the following competency:

Domain: Effective midwifery practice

- Complete, store and retain records of practice which:
  - are accurate, legible and continuous;
  - detail the reasoning behind any actions taken;
  - contain the information necessary for the record's purpose.

Chapter aims

After reading this chapter, you will be able to:

- define a health record;
- outline the two purposes of a health record;
- describe what must be included in a record entry;
- discuss the elements of good record keeping;
- understand the role of auditing in raising the standard of record keeping;
- compare and contrast the right of access to records of patients who are living with access to the records of patients who have died.

Introduction

In this chapter the importance of accurate record keeping to the safety of women and babies and its role in protecting midwives are considered. The legal implications of records are explained and we discuss how you should write records to ensure that the legal requirements are met. By drawing on case law, the chapter highlights the consequences for you of failing to meet those requirements.

Record keeping is a key aspect of a midwife's duty. The NMC considers that failing in this duty is professional misconduct of a type that can lead to the midwife being given a caution or suspension, or being removed from the professional register. The regulatory body has issued new guidelines on record keeping, effective from August 2009 (NMC, 2009d).

> CASE STUDY: Poor record keeping
>
> A registered midwife had her name removed from the professional register for poor record keeping. The midwife had failed to record the foetal heart rate as well as the maternal pulse that was required every 15 minutes in accordance with Trust policy. She failed to record any observations on a partogram and there were inconsistent entries in the clinical notes. (NMC Conduct and Competence Committee panel decision, 10 March 2010.)

What is a health record?

A health record is any electronic or paper information recorded about a person for the purpose of managing their healthcare (Data Protection Act 1998, s68(1)(a)). Health records include a variety of patient records that are held or filed within a hospital or GP practice. In midwifery it would include the community midwife's records, the hospital records, the child health record and X-rays, pathology reports, outpatients' reports, pharmacy records, etc. Together they form a record of the care and treatment a woman and her baby have received. Midwives are expected to keep detailed records of the care given to a woman throughout antenatal, intranatal and postnatal periods of pregnancy. For example, in 2009, a midwife was suspended for a year following her failure to document the care of a number of women in her care. She failed, among other things, to record observations made concerning blood transfusions, intravenous fluids and blood pressure monitoring (NMC, 2009f).

> Activity 8.1   Reflection
>
> • Why do you believe that the NMC regards record keeping as such an important duty?
> • Write down what you consider to be the purpose of keeping records.
>
> *Please do not move on to the next part until you are ready for the answer.*

The purpose of record keeping

The primary purpose of keeping records is to have an account of the care and treatment given to a patient. This allows progress to be monitored and a clinical history to be developed. The clinical record allows for continuity of care by facilitating care, treatment and support. The NMC emphasises that record keeping is not an optional extra to be fitted in when circumstances allow, but an integral part of care that is every bit as important as the direct care provided to women and their babies (NMC, 2009d).

As well as their clinical function, records have a very important legal purpose. They provide evidence of your involvement with a patient and they therefore need to be sufficiently detailed to demonstrate this involvement.

CASE STUDY: The legal function of records

In *S (A Child) v Newcastle & North Tyneside HA* [2001], the negligent mismanagement of the latter stages of labour resulted in severe cerebral palsy. The judge's annoyance at the poor standard of record keeping is clear from his judgment, where he comments on the lack of evidence in the records and partogram, making them devoid of any useful information.

The standard of proof in civil cases is the balance of probability – that is, if the weight of evidence is 51 per cent in your favour the case is won. As a midwife, your contact with women is mainly on a one-to-one basis, so it is your word against that of the mother. Records made at the time of, or soon after, seeing a mother often provide the necessary evidence to tip the case in your favour. For example, in *McLennan v Newcastle HA* [1992], a woman claimed she had not been told of the relatively high risk of failure associated with her sterilisation operation. The surgeon, however, had written in the notes at the time that the risks were explained and understood by the woman. This contemporaneous record persuaded the judge that she had probably been told about the risks and the case failed.

Legal implications of records

The Data Protection Act 1998 defines a health record very widely. In litigation that definition becomes wider still. The discovery process of a case allows any material document to be used as evidence. Any document that records any aspect of care can be required as evidence before a court of law or before any of the regulatory bodies. There is no restriction on access to these documents. The rules of the court demand that all documents are produced (Supreme Court Rules, Order 24). It is important, therefore, that midwives do not view record keeping as a mechanistic process. What you write does matter. In litigation the outcome is not based on truth but proof. If it is not in the notes it can be difficult to prove it happened. Cases are won and lost on the strength of records.

Next time you write in notes remember that you may be relying on them as evidence in court. They are of little value to you if they do not contain the information necessary to demonstrate that you have discharged your duty of care with professional skill and diligence. Records are never neutral; they will either support or condemn you.

Activity 8.2   *Reflection*

Write down the information you feel needs to be contained in a woman's midwifery record.

Please do not move on to the next part until you are ready for the answer.

What to include

Midwives have a statutory duty to maintain detailed records. The *Midwives Rules and Standards* set out the midwife's legal obligations in relation to record keeping.

Concept summary: Record keeping requirements for midwives

Rule 9 of the *Midwives Rules and Standards* (NMC, 2004b) states the following.

A practising midwife shall keep, as contemporaneously as is reasonable, continuous and detailed records of observations made, care given and medicine and any form of pain relief administered by her to a woman or baby.
   The records shall be kept:

a) in the case of a midwife employed by an NHS authority, in accordance with any directions given by her employer;
b) in any other case, in a form approved by the local supervising authority covering her main area of practice.

A midwife must not destroy or permit the destruction of records which have been made whilst she is in attendance upon a woman or baby.
   Immediately before ceasing to practise or if she finds it impossible or inconvenient to preserve her records safely, a midwife shall transfer them:

a) if she is employed by an NHS authority, to that authority;
b) if she is employed by a private sector employer, to that employer;
c) if she is not covered by paragraph (a) or (b), to the local supervising authority in whose area the care took place.

Any transfer must be duly recorded by each party to the transfer.

The requirements of this rule mean that your records need to be sufficiently detailed to show you have discharged your duty of care. An evidence-based care plan and regular progress reports form the backbone of this detail. To be useful in evidence, however, the record needs to show much more. Midwives often make 'wait and see' decisions. Should a woman be referred to hospital now or shall I wait and see? These wait and see decisions and the rationale behind them must be recorded so that a court, conduct committee or supervisor can see the reasoning behind your decision.

CASE STUDY: Delay in delivery

In *L v West Midlands SHA* [2009], a baby sued after suffering brain damage as a result of cord occlusion at the end of labour. It was agreed between the parties that, had the baby been delivered earlier, he would have suffered no brain damage. The court had to determine whether the midwives had called for an obstetrician promptly and whether the doctor had responded in time.
   The court decided that, although the midwives did not call for assistance immediately, they did call for a doctor when they were unable to confirm foetal well-being and had recorded evidence to indicate that the baby's condition was deteriorating. The court decided that the midwives had called for an obstetrician at the correct time and had not breached their duty of care. The obstetrician, however, did not respond quickly enough in the court's view and had been negligent.

The case study above shows how crucial it is to include care decisions in the woman's record. If you decide that a particular form of treatment or care should be delayed, say so. If you decide to wait and see before you call for a doctor or other assistance, record why you decided to wait.

Decisions about care and treatment are often taken on a multidisciplinary basis. Your records must include the background to the discussion and its outcome. This will indicate the reason for the decision and corroborate the account of other team members. Records must also corroborate any legal requirement or form completed by the woman in your presence. For example, if a woman signs a consent form, that should be recorded and the details discussed included. Details of telephone calls made, even if unanswered, to the woman or to others about the woman or her baby and discussions arising from them, with date and time, should be included, as should referrals to specialist practitioners. Where there are particular concerns, these telephone conversations should be confirmed in a letter. The importance of this measure is well illustrated by the following case study.

CASE STUDY: Victoria Climbié inquiry

Victoria Climbié died as a result of systematic abuse by her aunt. An inquiry into her death focused on the transfer of the case from a neighbouring social services department (DH, 2003c). The social worker assigned to her case told the inquiry that she had contacted the social services department, who told her the family had moved out of the borough, so the case was closed.

Social services denied the conversation took place and the department was still seeing Victoria and her aunt in December 1999, fully four months after she was referred.

The social worker admitted that she could not remember exactly when the phone conversation had taken place, nor had she dated the entry about the phone call in the files.

The Royal College of Midwives (RCM, 2005) has stressed that the lessons from the Victoria Climbié case are as pertinent to midwives as to agencies dealing with older children. For example, a father was found guilty of killing his six-week-old baby daughter who had suffered brain damage and a fractured skull (Ballinger, 2010). The baby had been seen by a midwife and a health visitor who reported that her condition had not caused concern. In the 24 days leading up to the 999 call she had not seen any professionals. The prosecutor in the case stated that the baby had been failed by the very people she should have been able to rely on.

Team members occasionally have differences of opinion on patient care. Any expression of dissent you have with another midwife, doctor or pharmacist should be recorded and the facts leading to the disagreement, the reason why you object and, importantly, what follow-up action was taken should be included.

Views of women and relatives

A further essential entry must be the views of women and their relatives. It is useful to differentiate the views of patients and relatives and your own entry by using quotation marks, for example 'I'm in agony with the pain.' Relatives or partners are an important source of progress or concern about women in your care. They know the woman well and notice changes in condition more quickly as a result. Their views must be recorded and responded to.

Scenario

Mary opted for a home birth. Her husband Mark was concerned about the level of anxiety his wife was exhibiting. He phoned Jane, the midwife assigned to support Mary at home, expressing concerns about his wife's behaviour. Jane reassured Mark that it was normal for pregnant women to exhibit some anxiety at the imminent arrival of the baby, but promised to pop in on her way home.

A few hours later Mark, alarmed at his wife's behaviour, phoned Jane again but could not reach her. He phoned the midwifery unit for advice. They told him that Jane would be calling on her way home and not to worry. Two hours later Mark found Mary attempting to cut her wrists. He called for an ambulance and she was transferred to the hospital.

Mark has complained at the lack of support given to him and his wife. A review by the supervisor of midwives found that the notes made no reference to the phone calls or advice given to Mark and were in breach of the *Midwives Rules and Standards* (NMC, 2004b), the NMC *Code* (2008a) and the NMC guidelines for record keeping (2009d), which state that midwives must record details of any assessments and reviews undertaken and provide clear evidence of the arrangements made for future and ongoing care. This should also include details of information given about care and treatment. The case was referred to the NMC preliminary proceedings committee for consideration of professional misconduct.

Records must be legible

It is essential that all records, instructions, prescriptions or referrals be written legibly and indelibly. Records are the key tool of communication between midwives. It is essential that record entries can be read. This begins with the clarity of the entry. Clarity requires ink that contrasts with the paper being used for entries, with white paper and black ink giving the greatest contrast and best clarity when copied. In litigation a record will be copied to each of the relevant parties. That means that, on average, some 20 copies will be made. Records are of little use as evidence if the writing cannot be read due to deterioration in clarity when photocopied.

The standard of your handwriting is also a requirement of your duty of care to a patient. If care is initiated by you through a care plan and harm results because others could not read your writing, liability in negligence is likely to arise. This is illustrated in the following key case study.

CASE STUDY: A doctor with poor handwriting

In *Prendergast v Sam and Dee Ltd* [1989], an illegible prescription for Amoxil resulted in a man being given the wrong drug, Daonil, which caused hypoglycaemia and brain damage. The pharmacist was found to be 75 per cent liable for that harm for dispensing the wrong drug. For his poor handwriting the GP was found to be 25 per cent liable. The Court of Appeal held that there is a duty to write clearly enough for a busy or careless person to read your instructions.

Legibility extends to the signature of the person who made the entry. Identifying the people and, therefore, witnesses involved in an incident is crucial to building a successful case. As well as a signature, the name in print or block capitals and grade of the person writing should be noted at least once in the notes during the course of the record.

Writing with indelible ink or typeface is essential for two reasons. First, the records must stand the test of time. It may be many years before they are referred to again and a faded record is of little value as evidence. It is usual for several years to pass before an incident goes to court to be decided. Cases involving babies can take 21 years to come to court. It is essential that these records are available and their contents remain legible. The *Midwives Rules and Standards* (NMC, 2004b) require midwives to keep the records that relate to the women and babies in their care for at least 25 years.

CASE STUDY: 21 years for a case to come to court

In *Reynolds v North Tyneside HA* [2002], a woman argued that she had suffered cerebral palsy as a result of the negligent mismanagement of her mother's labour some 21 years earlier. The patient's records and hospital policy were central to the case. In this instance, the patient's records were in good condition and properly completed. They showed that staff attending the birth had acted according to hospital policy. It was the hospital policy that was found to be incorrect and the court found for the woman.

The credibility of your record as evidence is enhanced by its being made at the time of the incident. Credibility is essential to the reliability of the record as evidence of what occurred. Using indelible ink or typeface reassures the court that the entry has not been subsequently altered in any way. You must therefore avoid using pencil or a computer entry system that does not use a time stamp or some other method to ensure that the entry cannot be altered without a trace. Altering a record is seen as a serious matter and can result in prosecution, dismissal and removal from the nursing register as the following case study shows.

CASE STUDY: Student who altered record is jailed

A student who faked her birth delivery figures to boost her hopes of qualifying as a midwife was jailed for six months (Hampshire and Isle of Wight Counter Fraud Team, 2007). The student altered computer records at the hospital to show she had gained sufficient experience to qualify in her profession. Using colleagues' passwords, she changed the details to convince her supervisor that she had overseen almost 30 births more than she actually had.

Records must be clear and unambiguous

Records are an essential tool in the continuity of care. Care to be implemented and progress made must be clearly stated. The record is also likely to be read by people other than midwives. Child health records are often left with parents, and a woman has a right to access her records under the Data Protection Act 1998. The Human Rights Act 1998 (schedule 1, part 1, article 8) gives a separate right of access for women and, in some respects, relatives where this affects their right to respect for a private and family life. In *Gaskin v UK* [1990], the European Court of Human Rights emphasised the need for specific justification for preventing individuals from having access to information that forms part of their private and family life.

Ownership of records

The Secretary of State technically owns a woman's NHS records, except where the midwife is self-employed, but normally delegates this responsibility to individual Trusts and health authorities. The records are not owned by the person who completes them. Therefore, midwives need to have a good understanding of what amounts to a health record. For example, clinical entries relating to a named patient in a diary may be a health record and the diaries cannot be discarded or destroyed. Where the midwife ceases to practise, such records need to be returned to the relevant Trust, health authority, private sector employer or to the local supervising authority if the midwife is self-employed (NMC, 2004b). In addition, rule 10 of the *Midwives Rules and Standards* provides that practising midwives must allow a supervisor of midwives, a local supervising authority and the NMC to monitor their standards and methods of practice and to inspect their records, equipment and any premises that they use for professional purposes. That may include the midwife's home.

The self-employed midwife

Self-employed midwives own their records and must preserve the records of all their clients and keep them in a safe place. In addition, independent midwives must transfer the records to the local supervisory authority when they cease to practise.

Access to health records

A legal right of access to health records is given to living people whether their records are computerised or manually created (handwritten) under the provisions of the Data Protection Act 1998 and its regulations. The right of access applies equally to all records regardless of when they were made. Limited statutory rights of access to the records of deceased patients still exist in the Access to Health Records Act 1990.

Access rights under the Data Protection Act 1998

Patients have a right to be informed when personal data about them is being processed (this includes obtaining, recording or holding information and why; for more detail, see Chapter 9).

Women have a right of access to health records that:

- are about them and from which they can be identified;
- consist of information relating to their physical or mental health or condition;
- have been made by or on behalf of a health professional in connection with their care.

Where access is agreed, the health record must be communicated to the woman in an intelligible form. That will often require the midwife responsible for the record meeting the woman to explain the content and any technical or cryptic remarks or abbreviations that may be within it. A woman is entitled to a permanent copy of the information and this must also be accompanied by an explanation of any terms that are unintelligible. Where the woman considers that the record or part of it is inaccurate, she can seek a correction.

You are not obliged to accept the woman's opinion or version of events, but you must ensure that the record indicates her view and provide a copy of the correction or appended note. These arrangements must indicate why the alteration was made to avoid any allegation of tampering with the record.

If the woman remains dissatisfied with her record, she may take the matter to court. The courts have the power to insist that inaccurate data and any expression of opinion based on them are corrected or removed. The court may also require the records to be supplemented by a statement of the true facts, and third parties to be notified of any corrections.

Applications for access

Nothing in the 1998 Act prevents you from giving women access to their records on an informal and voluntary basis, provided no other provisions of the Act preventing disclosure are breached. Indeed, the Data Protection Act 1998 calls for you to work in partnership with women in an open and informal way so that, if access to a record is requested, there are no surprises. Formal applications for access must be in writing and accompanied by the appropriate fee.

Anyone is entitled to seek access to their health records. In the case of a child, any person with parental responsibility may apply, independently. Where the child's parents live apart and have parental responsibility, they may individually apply to see their child's record. The other parent does not need to be told.

In *Gillick v West Norfolk and Wisbech AHA* [1986], the House of Lords held that, where children are competent to make their own decisions about treatment, they are entitled to the same degree of confidentiality as an adult patient. Where access to a competent child's record is requested, it can only be granted if the child consents (see Chapter 6).

Competent children and young people may, of course, seek access to their own health records, and anyone can authorise a third party, such as a relative or legal representative, to seek access on their behalf.

Requests for access are made to the person in charge of keeping the records, known under the Data Protection Act 1998 as the data controller. The decision about disclosure is made by the appropriate health professional. This person would be the health professional currently or most recently responsible for the care of the woman. Access must be given promptly and, in any event, within 40 days of receipt of the fee and clear request. Where access is given, there is no obligation to give access again until a reasonable time interval has elapsed. There is no legal guidance on how long this would be and it must be assessed on a case by case basis. For example, if the patient has received no further treatment in the intervening period, a grant of access would seem unreasonable.

Information that cannot be disclosed

The right of access does not include information that would identify some other person mentioned in the record. This information cannot be released unless:

- the third party is a health professional who has compiled or contributed to the health records or who has been involved in the care of the patient;
- the other individual gives consent to the disclosure of that information; or
- it is reasonable to dispense with that third party's consent.

Where the record includes information from other identifiable sources, it is advisable to distinguish this information in the records when the information is entered in order to avoid inadvertent disclosure. It is still necessary to disclose as much of the information in the records as is possible, but you must ensure that you:

- omit names and identifying particulars from the records before disclosure;
- ensure that the information is genuinely anonymous.

You are not obliged to approach a third party for consent to disclosure, although you may wish to in some circumstances.

Harm

Access must not be given to any information that, in the opinion of the appropriate health professional, would be likely to cause serious harm to the patient or another person.

This exemption does not justify withholding comments in the records because women may find them upsetting. For example, in *R (on the application of S) v Plymouth City Council* [2002], a mother was refused access to her vulnerable son's health and social services record. She argued that she needed access to help her make decisions about his future. The court granted access and it then emerged that the record contained uncomplimentary remarks about the woman.

Children

The Data Protection Act 1998 does not allow disclosure of information prohibited in legislation concerning adoption records and reports, statements of a child's special educational needs and parental order records and reports. None of these exemptions apply where the disclosure is required by law, or is necessary for the purposes of establishing, exercising or defending legal rights.

Access to records of deceased people

The Data Protection Act 1998 does not cover the records of deceased people. Statutory rights of access are granted within the provisions of the Access to Health Records Act 1990.

Any person with a claim arising from the death of a person has a right of access to information covered by the Act in cases where this information is directly relevant to that claim. The information that can be accessed is, however, restricted to that covered by the Act, that is, manually created (handwritten) health records made since 1 November 1991.

The quality of records

Use of jargon and abbreviations

Activity 8.3   **Group work**

- Write down a list of abbreviations and technical jargon you have used or read during your clinical placements.
- Now pass the lists among your colleagues and ask them to explain what they understand by the terms and abbreviations.
- Did you all come to the same definitions and meanings of the terms?

As the answer will be based on your own experiences, there is no outline answer at the end of the chapter.

The temptation to use jargon and abbreviations as a form of professional shorthand is compelling for busy, overworked midwives. However, the risk of miscommunication increases dramatically in using this shorthand.

> ### CASE STUDY: Poor handwriting and abbreviations
>
> Diabetes is an increasingly common disorder and one that can affect the health of women and their babies. Insulin is often required to manage the disease, but a study of prescriptions (Cox and Ferner, 2009) has shown that poor handwriting caused an unacceptably high percentage of errors and a misunderstanding of an abbreviation for insulin units had serious consequences for several women who suffered hypoglycaemic episodes.

Although under considerable work pressure, midwives must not use abbreviations or jargon. The risks are too great and misinterpretation by staff is common.

Jargon is also used to convey offensive remarks unrelated to patient care. Offensive cryptic acronyms include CLL (chronic low life), FLK (funny looking kid), often explained by JLD (just like dad).

Remember that, in litigation, your records will be subjected to rigorous scrutiny. You have no right to withhold any part of the record from the court. Having to explain under cross-examination that the entry GLM meant that you thought the woman was a 'glum-looking mum' or that LOBNH meant 'lights on but nobody home' will be at best embarrassing and at worst fatal to your case. Evidentially, the first impression the court has of you is from your notes. If your records are not professional, the assumption is that neither is your care and your credibility as a witness is greatly diminished.

Records must be accurate

To confirm the chronology of record entries, each entry must be identified with the date (day, month and year) and time (using the 24-hour clock) and signed, with the midwife's name printed legibly underneath the signature together with his or her position. Initials for entries must not be used as it is vital to be able to identify the member of staff if a complaint is made.

> ### CASE STUDY: Ten minutes of unexplained delay
>
> In *Richards v Swansea NHS Trust* [2007], a baby suffered cerebral palsy and it was argued that it was as the result of a delayed emergency caesarean. The operation occurred some 50 minutes after it was considered necessary. Professional guidance stated that it must occur within 30 minutes and the judge was content to grant the Trust a period of 40 minutes, but the Trust and care team had to justify the extra 10-minute delay. As they were unable to produce records to demonstrate what call on their time there was during that 10-minute period, the judge said he had no alternative but to find them negligent.

Errors

All alterations must be made by scoring out with a single line that does not completely obscure the error. Correcting fluid must not be used. This removes any suggestion of wrongdoing or attempting to cover up an incident. The struck-out error should be followed by the dated, timed and signed correct entry. No blank lines or spaces that could facilitate entries being added at a later date should be left between entries.

Pressure of work

It may be argued that pressure of work was such that it reduced the midwife's ability to maintain the usual standard of care. Such situations have been called battlefield situations, in which resources are so stretched that a court has to accept that the expected level of the standard of care must be reduced (*Wilsher v Essex HA* [1988]). In these situations the court can order the disclosure of other patients' records to see how busy the ward was.

CASE STUDY: Pressure of work

In *Deacon v McVicar* (1984), a woman argued that she had received negligent care causing her harm. The hospital argued that the evening of the incident was a singularly busy one, with several emergency cases draining available resources. The court ordered that the records of all other patients on the ward that evening be released to the court to see how busy the unit was. They showed that it was an exceptionally busy evening, with many emergencies overstretching the staff and resources. No more could have been expected of the staff and they were not negligent.

Contemporaneous record entries

Record entries need to be written at the time of, or as soon as possible after, the events to which they relate. Contemporaneous recording is vital as it adds to the reliability of the entry and means that, with the leave of the court, you can refer to the record when giving evidence. Contemporaneous altering of a record contributed to a finding of negligence in *Kent v Griffiths and Others* [2000]. Here, an emergency ambulance took 30 minutes to arrive at an address, but the crew recorded the duration of the journey as nine minutes. The judge held that the record had been contemporaneously falsified and found for the patient.

The record should demonstrate the chronology of events and of all significant consultations, assessments, observations, decisions, interventions and outcomes. Reports and results should be seen, evaluated and signed by the practitioner before being filed in the patient records. This is the key to a good record. This is what a lawyer is going to try to pull apart in order to win a case.

Records are never neutral

To be of use in evidence your records need to be thorough, otherwise they will act to your detriment. Records are never neutral; they will either support you or condemn you.

CASE STUDY: The incomplete record

In *S (A Child) v Newcastle and North Tyneside HA* [2001], the negligent management of the latter stages of labour resulted in severe cerebral palsy. The judge's annoyance at the standard of record keeping is clear from his comments:

It is important to emphasise at this early stage that unhappily the evidence was, in certain important respects, incomplete. The clinical records of this labour are not full and no records at all appear between 4 a.m. and 10.15 a.m. Each of these might be regarded as critical periods.

Unhappily whoever did take over from [the midwife] singularly failed to complete the partogram, that is the record of the labour, which is effectively devoid of useful information.

The importance of personal details

The woman's and her baby's personal details are every bit as important as the care plan and progress entries. The Audit Commission (1999) found that the average NHS Trust wastes some £20,000 per year on redirected mail, due to incorrect home addresses or GP details that have been recorded in the notes or on the computer system. Missing details also reduce the quality of care by disrupting communication between women, their families and health staff, causing missed appointments and losing potentially critical information. It is important to check details with women to ensure that personal information is up to date.

Keeping records secure

All NHS records are public records under the provisions of the Public Records Act 1958, section 3. The Secretary of State for Health and all NHS organisations have a duty under this Act to make arrangements for the safekeeping and eventual disposal of all records. Chief executives and senior managers of all NHS organisations are personally account-able for the safekeeping of records.

Activity 8.4 *Critical thinking*

What measures must you take to ensure the safety and security of patient records?

Please do not move on to the next part until you are ready for the answer.

Under the Public Records Act 1958, midwives are accountable for any records that they create or use in the course of their duties. You have a duty to ensure that records are kept safe and secure by:

- ensuring the physical security of such records, keeping records locked away when not required;
- ensuring that records and their binders are in a good state so that information is held securely, loose-leaf information such as test results is properly secured, and information cannot be lost or mislaid from the record;
- maintaining security of access to information within the records by ensuring that they cannot be inadvertently read by others;
- maintaining a written log of incoming/outgoing records through the use of a tracing system that allows for the physical tracking of records.

Putting the record straight

The Audit Commission (1999) found that subjecting records to a regular audit is the best way to ensure high-quality record keeping. Employers can determine how and when midwifery records made by midwives employed by them are audited. Independent midwives have a duty to protect their client's information and they should ensure that such notes are only available for audit purposes with the permission of the client.

Activity 8.5   *Reflection*

Having read this chapter, if you were to audit your record entries, what key standards would you wish to meet?

Please do not move on to the next part until you are ready for the answer.

In an advice sheet on record keeping, the NMC (2007) recommends the following content for healthcare records.

Patient records must be:

- factual, consistent and accurate;
- written in such a way that the meaning is clear;
- recorded as soon as possible after an event has occurred;
- recorded clearly and indelibly;
- recorded so that any justifiable alterations or additions are dated, timed and signed in such a way that the original entry can still be read clearly;
- accurately dated, timed and signed, with the signature printed alongside the first entry where this is a written record, and attributed to a named person in an identifiable role for electronic records;
- free from abbreviations, jargon, meaningless phrases, irrelevant speculation, offensive or subjective statements;
- readable when photocopied or scanned;
- recorded, wherever possible, with the involvement of the patient;
- recorded in terms that the patient can understand;
- in chronological order;
- specific about risks or problems that have arisen and the action taken to rectify them;
- clear and accurate about the assessment and the care that has been planned and provided;
- able to provide relevant information about the condition of the patient;
- able to provide evidence that you have discharged your duty of care;
- able to provide a record of any arrangements that have been made for the continuing care of a patient.

You are also required to make more frequent entries for women who:

- have complex problems;
- are vulnerable or at risk of harm or abuse;
- require more intensive care than normal;
- are confused and disoriented or generally give cause for concern.

C H A P T E R   S U M M A R Y

- Records are a fundamental aspect of a midwife's duty towards the women in his or her care. They provide a plan of care and are crucial in monitoring progress and communicating concerns.
- Records also provide evidence of involvement with women and babies.
- Records must be thorough, contemporaneous and clear, and must be communicated to be effective. Expressions of dissent must be recorded, and records must corroborate discussions with colleagues. Subjecting records to audit creates a higher standard of record keeping.
- Records have a vital role in protecting midwives from litigation. If an occurrence is not written down it is difficult to prove it happened. Thorough, contemporaneous, legible records will protect you from litigation by providing robust evidence of your involvement with a patient.
- In this way, you will demonstrate you have met your legal and professional obligations and discharged your duty of care.

Knowledge review

Having completed the chapter, how would you now rate your knowledge of the following topics?

	Good	Adequate	Poor
1. Defining a health record.			
2. The purposes of keeping records.			
3. The style and content of a midwifery record.			
4. The elements of good record keeping.			
5. Patients' rights of access to records.			

Where you're not confident in your knowledge of a topic, what will you do next?

Further reading

For key advice on record keeping in the context of healthcare see:

Department of Health (DH) (2006) *Records Management: NHS code of practice.* London: The Stationery Office.

Nursing and Midwifery Council (NMC) (2009) *Record Keeping: Guidance for nurses and midwives.* London: NMC.

For a consideration of the common problems associated with poor records, we recommend you read:

Audit Commission (1999) *Setting the Record Straight: A review of progress in health records services.* London: The Stationery Office.

Useful websites

www.library.nhs.uk/Default.aspx NHS Evidence, which is an excellent website that has a searchable database of guidelines and standards, including those for record keeping.

www.nmc-uk.org Nursing and Midwifery Council, which has guidance, advice and case studies on record keeping.

Chapter 9

Confidentiality

NMC Standards for Pre-registration Midwifery Education

This chapter will address the following competency:

Domain: Professional and ethical practice
- Maintain confidentiality of information. This will include:
    - ensuring the confidentiality and security of written and verbal information acquired in a professional capacity;
    - disclosing information about individuals and organisations only to those who have a right and need to know this information, and only once proof of identity and right to disclosure has been obtained.

Chapter aims

After reading this chapter, you will be able to:
- discuss the rationale for imposing a duty of confidence on registered midwives;
- outline three spheres of the duty of confidence that registered midwives are subject to;
- compare the scope of the legal, professional and contractual obligation of confidence;
- describe the circumstances that would allow you to disclose confidential information;
- explain three ways in which the duty of confidence may be modified by statute;
- discuss the measures midwives must take to ensure that confidential information is disclosed with appropriate care.

Introduction

This chapter explores confidentiality in the context of midwifery care. It considers the scope and sources of a midwife's duty of confidentiality, before discussing the circumstances that would allow you to disclose information relating to a woman or her baby. The chapter then highlights the measures you must take to ensure that any disclosure of information is done with appropriate care.

Maintaining the confidentiality of health information is a fundamental element of professional conduct and ethical practice for all registered midwives. The relationship between the midwife and mother is essential for proper assessment and care that is largely based on a woman's personal history of her health problems. Sensitive information about their health and other matters will be disclosed by women as part of their desire to receive the best care. They have a right to expect you to respect their privacy by ensuring the confidentiality of all the information they give.

To ensure the highest standard of conduct and ethical practice in relation to the protection of health information, a duty of confidence is imposed on all staff, volunteers and contractors within the NHS.

Activity 9.1   *Reflection*

Before you continue reading the chapter, write down what you understand by the term 'confidentiality'.

Please do not move on to the next part until you are ready for the answer.

Duty of confidence

A duty of confidence arises when one person discloses information to another in circumstances where it is reasonable to expect that the information will be held in confidence.

For midwives there are three key spheres to the duty that come together to reassure women that the confidentiality of their health information will be respected (see Figure 9.1).

1. A duty to respect confidentiality that is a specific requirement linked to disciplinary procedures in all NHS employment contracts and underpinned by the NHS code of practice on confidentiality (DH, 2003a).
2. A legal duty that is derived from case law and supplemented by statute law (*Cornelius v De Taranto* [2001]).
3. A professional duty established by the NMC's *Code* (2008a).

However, the duty of confidence is not absolute. There will be occasions where confidential information will need to be disclosed to others. Such a disclosure must be to an appropriate person and comply with the requirements of your contractual, professional and legal duty of confidence or you will be called to account and face sanctions for breaching confidentiality.

It is essential, therefore, that you:

- understand the scope of the duty of confidence owed to the women in your care;
- only disclose information given in confidence where it is right and proper to do so.

Figure 9.1: The three spheres of the duty of confidence owed by registered midwives

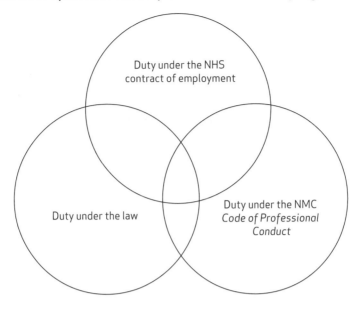

The scope of the duty

The contractual duty of confidence

In recognition of the need to protect women and maintain the confidentiality of health information, all contracts of employment in the NHS must contain a clause imposing a duty of confidence on all staff that stresses that disciplinary action will result if that duty is breached (DH, 2003a). Similarly, all contracts with outside agencies and arrangements with volunteers and others – including student midwives – who undertake work or placements with the NHS must also include a clause imposing a duty of confidence.

In order to discharge this duty, all staff and students will need to show that they have fulfilled their responsibilities by ensuring that they comply with the following.

• They must not disclose confidential information through inappropriate means such as gossiping.
• They must take care when discussing cases in their assignments. Matters relating to mothers and their babies must be anonymised in such a way that they cannot be identified through special features such as a specific birthmark or unique circumstances surrounding the birth of the child.

- When they seek advice about care and treatment from a colleague, they must do so in private so that confidentiality is not inadvertently breached.
- They must accurately record information received from and about women and their babies.
- They must keep information and records private and physically secure.
- They must only access information for the women in their care.
- They must only disclose information about a woman or baby to an appropriate source in accordance with the NHS code of practice on confidentiality, the requirements of the law and their code of professional conduct.

The following case study highlights the consequences of unjustified access and disclosure of health information for all health professionals and staff working in the NHS.

CASE STUDY: Celebrity records

When a former England manager was admitted to hospital to have surgery, his records were accessed by staff who were not involved in his clinical care but were curious to find out about their footballing hero (*Northern Echo*, 2006).

Officials at the Trust became suspicious when security reports showed that there had been inappropriate access to the Trust's patient records system.

Staff are not permitted to look up patient records unless there is a direct medical need. Disciplinary action was taken against ten members of staff at the hospital.

The duty to maintain confidentiality extends to all those who have received maternity services, both past and present. Although there is no specific legal or professional requirement that states that a duty of confidence extends to people who have died, the contractual duty imposed by the NHS extends confidentiality beyond the grave and does include the deceased.

The professional duty of confidence

The professional requirement for confidentiality is stipulated in the NMC's *Code* (2008a). This states that registered midwives must guard against breaches of confidentiality by protecting information from improper disclosure at all times.

Activity 9.3   *Research*

- Download and read the NMC's explanatory paper on confidentiality (2008; available at **www.nmc-uk.org/Nurses-and-midwives/Advice-by-topic/A/ Advice/Confidentiality**).
- Then outline the extent of a midwife's professional duty of confidence to patients.
- List the exceptions to that duty that would allow you to disclose information about a patient.

Please do not move on to the next part until you are ready for the answer.

This professional duty imposes on midwives a requirement not voluntarily to disclose information gained in a professional capacity to a third party. This duty is enforced by the threat of professional discipline. An explanatory paper by the NMC on professional conduct highlights a breach of confidentiality as a form of misconduct likely to result in removal from the register, as shown in the following case study (NMC, 2004c).

CASE STUDY: Inappropriate disclosure of patient information

A specialist community public health practitioner who had an affair with an ex-patient told him of an abortion his partner had undergone 19 years earlier (*Evening Gazette*, 2006). When asked where she had got the information from, she revealed that it had come from the woman's health record. The health practitioner admitted breaching confidentiality and was found guilty by a professional competence and conduct committee of the NMC, which removed her name from the professional register.

The duty of confidence and the law

As well as the professional duty of confidence there is a legal obligation on midwives to respect the confidences of the women and babies in their care. The law relating to confidence is dealt with largely at common law. The obligation arises out of a general duty on everyone to keep confidential information secret (*Prince Albert v Strange* (1849)) – that is, there is a public interest in keeping confidential information secret.

In order to establish a breach of confidence, three elements must be satisfied, as stated by the House of Lords in *Attorney General v Guardian Newspapers* [1988]:

1. The information must have the necessary quality of confidence – that is, the information is not generally available or known. Information of a personal or intimate nature qualifies (*Stephens v Avery* [1988]), and this is very much the type of information you receive from the women in your care.
2. The information must be imparted in circumstances giving rise to an obligation of confidence. The law has long recognised that particular relationships give rise to a duty of confidence. These include the relationships of priest and penitent, solicitor and client, and midwife and mother. The courts have gone further, however, extending the obligation to include situations where an obviously confidential document is wafted by an electric fan out of a window into a crowded street, where a private diary is dropped in a public place, or even when an email goes astray.
3. The information must be divulged to a third person without the permission and to the detriment of the person originally communicating the information. An invasion of personal privacy will suffice (*Margaret, Duchess of Argyll v Duke of Argyll* [1965]). As it is in the public interest that medical confidences are kept secret, the court will regard an unwarranted disclosure of patient information as detrimental (*Attorney General v Guardian (No. 2)* [1988] (Lord Keith)).

It can be seen that the very private nature of the information midwives are given by mothers, and the trust generated by the nature of the midwife–mother relationship, gives rise to an obligation of confidence that the law seeks to protect. Consequently, the court will consider that an inappropriate disclosure of this information is bound to be detrimental and find that a breach of confidence has occurred.

CASE STUDY: Breaching the common law duty of confidence

In *X v Y and Others* [1988], a health authority employee passed on to a newspaper information obtained from the medical records of two doctors who were HIV positive. The doctors worked in the area and the newspaper wished to publish the details. The court granted the doctors an injunction preventing publication, holding that the public interest in preserving the confidentiality of hospital records outweighed any public interest in the freedom of the press, because victims of the disease ought not to be deterred by fear of discovery from going to hospital for treatment.

As well as a general duty of confidence established under the common law, there is a range of statutory provisions that limit or prohibit the use and disclosure of information in specific circumstances.

Data Protection Act 1998

The Data Protection Act 1998 implements a European Union (EU) directive on the protection of individuals with regard to the processing of personal data and on the free movement of such data (Directive 95/46/EC). The Act provides a framework that governs the so-called processing of personal data.

Personal data is defined under the Act as data that relates to a living individual who can be identified either from that data, or from data and other information that may be in your possession. This includes any expression of opinion about the individual and any indications of your intentions towards the individual.

'Processing' is an umbrella term and includes:

- holding information about people;
- obtaining information from a person or others about a person;
- recording health information;
- using the information;
- disclosing health information.

The Act applies to all forms of media, including paper records, electronic records and images.

All processing of health information must be fair and lawful. This will usually be the case where:

- the common law of confidentiality and any other applicable statutory restrictions on the use of information are complied with;
- the mother, known as the data subject, was not misled or deceived into giving the information;
- the woman is given basic information about who will process the data and for what purpose;
- in the case of personal health information, the conditions of schedules 2 and 3 of the Data Protection Act 1998 concerning sensitive data are met by ensuring that the information is necessary for medical purposes.

Human Rights Act 1998

Article 8 of the European Convention on Human Rights 1950 establishes a right to respect for private and family life. This right emphasises the duty to protect the privacy of individuals and preserve the confidentiality of their health records. Article 8 is broad in scope and covers the collection, use and exchange of personal data, as well as issues such as telephone tapping, parental access and custody of children, the right to be free from noise and environmental pollution, and a person's right to express their identity and sexuality. Public authorities must preserve the individual's confidence when collecting and using personal data.

For example, in *R (Robertson) v City of Wakefield Metropolitan Council* [2002], a man complained that his right to respect for a private life under article 8 of the Convention was being infringed by his local council, as they were selling personal details he was required to provide for inclusion on the electoral roll to commercial companies. These companies were using the information for direct marketing.

The court held that article 8 was breached by the council. In determining whether article 8 was engaged, it was necessary to take into account not just the information that was disclosed, but also the use to which it would be put. Where names and addresses were to be passed on to commercial companies for direct marketing purposes, this amounted to an interference with the right to private life.

Exceptions to the obligation of confidence

Both the professional and legal duties of confidentiality are not absolute and are subject to a range of exceptions that justify disclosure. It is important that midwives are aware of these exceptions in order to avoid a charge of professional misconduct and liability for breach of confidence.

The NMC generally leaves the decision to divulge a confidence with the registered midwife by viewing it as a matter of professional judgement. Yet little specific guidance is given on circumstances where disclosure is justified. No guidance is given on the difference between a power to disclose, where a midwife can consider all the circumstances and decide if it is appropriate to divulge information; and a duty to disclose, where, regardless of circumstances, the law requires disclosure.

Activity 9.4	*Reflection*

The duty of confidence owed by the midwife is not absolute. There will be times when it will be appropriate to disclose information about a mother or her baby.

- Consider circumstances where you would think it was appropriate to divulge information about those in your care.

Please do not move on to the next part until you are ready for the answer.

Consent of the patient

Permission to disclose confidential information given by the person who originally imparted it is the starting presumption in law and an obvious exception. The courts generally require this consent to disclosure to be in the form of an explicit consent, preferably signed by the woman (*Cornelius v DeTaranto* [2001]). This ruling also reflects the requirements of the Data Protection Act 1998. The consent exception is only valid if the person knows exactly what information is to be disclosed and who is to receive the information.

The requirements for obtaining explicit consent from patients for the disclosure of personal health information are as follows.

- Be honest and clear about the information to be disclosed and the reason for disclosure, allowing women to seek as much detail as they require to make a free choice.
- Give women an opportunity to talk to someone they trust and to ask questions.
- Allow reasonable time to reach a decision.
- Be prepared to explain any form that may need to be signed.
- Explain that consent can be refused or withdrawn at any time.
- Ensure that you note that consent has been received in the health record or by using a consent form signed by the woman.

Disclosure for care and treatment purposes

An area where a midwife might exercise professional judgement and disclose confidential information is with those directly involved in the care of the mother and baby.

Confidentiality is allowed to be breached where information is shared with other midwives concerned with the clinical care of the mother and baby. This exception also covers doctors and others, where the information provided is necessary for the performance of their duties. These professionals are also bound by a duty of confidentiality. To require an express consent each time a case was discussed would be impractical and even detrimental.

Where women have consented to healthcare, research has consistently shown that they are content for information to be disclosed in order to provide that healthcare (NHSIA, 2002). It is still essential that you ensure that women understand how their information is to be used to support their healthcare and that they have no objections by adhering to the following guidelines.

- Check where practicable that information leaflets on confidentiality and information disclosure have been read and understood by the women in your care.
- Make it clear why personal health information is recorded and why health records need to be accessed by other health professionals.
- Make it clear why you need to share their health information with others.
- Ensure that women have no concerns about how you will use their personal information.
- Answer any questions that women may have or direct them to someone who can answer their questions.
- Respect the rights of women to request access to their health records.

If you have done all this, consent can be implied, provided that the information is shared no more widely than with those directly concerned with the care and treatment of the individual. Wide disclosure to any doctor or midwife is not justified, as can be seen from this case study.

CASE STUDY: Limits to the clinical family

In *Cornelius v De Taranto* [2001], a teacher who claimed to be suffering from work-related stress saw a psychiatrist privately as part of evidence gathering against her employer. The psychiatrist sent a copy of her medico-legal report to the teacher's GP and a general consultant psychiatrist, as well as to her solicitor. The teacher sued for breach of confidence. The Court of Appeal held that there was a breach of confidence as the report had nothing to do with her treatment, so dissemination to other health professionals could not be justified on therapeutic grounds.

Women who refuse consent to disclose treatment information

Women have the right to be informed that they can object to the disclosure of confidential information that identifies them. If a woman refuses to allow information to be disclosed to other health professionals involved in providing care, this might mean that the care provided will be limited. Women must be told if their refusal to allow disclosure of treatment information will have implications for the provision of care or treatment. Midwives cannot provide care safely or provide continuity of care without having relevant information about a woman's condition and medical history.

Disclosing information when a woman asks you to do so

If a woman asks you to pass on confidential information about her, the court regards this as a binding obligation. In *C v C* [1946], a judge considered the refusal of a sexually transmitted infection (STI) clinic to divulge information about a client despite their request for disclosure. The judge held that, while it was important that proper secrecy be observed in STI clinics, those considerations did not justify a health professional refusing to divulge confidential information to a named person when asked by the client so to do. In the circumstances of this case, the information should have been given, and in all cases where the circumstances are similar there is no breach of confidence in giving the information asked for. The following activity gives you an opportunity to explore further the views of service users on the disclosure of health information.

Activity 9.5   *Research and reflection*

- Download a copy of the NHS Information Authority's *Share with Care!: People's views on consent and confidentiality of patient information* (2002) at **www.connectingforhealth.nhs.uk/resources/archive/share_with_care.pdf**.
- Read and consider what the report discovered about service users' views on health professionals disclosing their personal information.

As this activity involves your own ideas and reflection, there is no outline answer at the end of the chapter.

Disclosing information without specific consent

There are a number of exceptions allowing disclosure to appropriate sources without consent (DH, 2003a). These exceptions act as a useful aid to midwives when making a judgement about disclosing information.

Where a woman is incapable of receiving information or of consenting to disclosure, disclosure of care and treatment information to the client's relative or main carer may be judged to be appropriate. Similarly, disclosure to appropriate sources would be allowed in cases of suspected abuse of a vulnerable woman or baby in accordance with vulnerable adult and child protection procedures as discussed in Chapters 7 and 11 (DH, 1999, 2002).

Disclosure in the public interest

A major defence used by individuals who have had to justify disclosure of confidential information has been that the disclosure was necessary in the public interest. The courts accept that, when a case concerning the disclosure of confidential information comes before them, they are required to strike a balance between two competing interests. The public interest in keeping confidential information secret must be weighed against the public interest in allowing disclosure.

The public interest exception covers a broad range of situations that allow for confidential information to be disclosed without consent. These situations include:

- disclosure in the interests of justice;
- disclosure for the public good;
- disclosure to protect a third party;
- disclosure to prevent or detect a serious crime.

Disclosure in the interests of justice

Unlike lawyers, midwives do not have a privileged relationship with the women in their care. A court has the power to order disclosure of confidential matters if it is in the interests of justice; refusing to do so would result in conviction for contempt of court. For example, in *Attorney General v Mulholland* [1963], two journalists refused before a tribunal to name or describe the sources of information in articles written by them. One of the journalists was sentenced to six and the other to three months' imprisonment for contempt.

In exercising this power the court must be satisfied that disclosure will satisfy the interests of justice. Where this is not the case they can refuse to order disclosure, as shown by the following case study.

CASE STUDY: Court refuses to order disclosure

In *D v National Society for the Prevention of Cruelty to Children* [1977], the NSPCC received a complaint from an informant about the alleged maltreatment of a girl aged 14 months. An inspector from the society called at the parents' home and inquired about the baby. The mother, who was very upset, called the family doctor, who found the baby to be healthy and unharmed. The family demanded to be told the name of the informant. When the inspector refused, they brought legal proceedings to reveal the identity of the informant. The House of Lords held that the public interest in preserving confidentiality of informants for the protection of children overrode the requirement that the mother should be given the information she sought to pursue her claim.

Midwives, therefore, could be required by the courts to disclose information about their patients, in the form of both written statements and oral evidence, where this is necessary in the interests of justice.

Disclosure for the public good

There may be circumstances where the public interest is served by disclosing information even though no crime has been committed or court action taken. This might include disclosing information to a regulatory body such as the NMC. Health professionals who come to the attention of the police, for example, will have their details passed on to their regulatory body, without it being considered a breach of confidence, if their fitness to practise is in question, as illustrated by the following case study.

CASE STUDY: No breach where fitness to practise is in question

In *Lancashire CC v W (A Child) (Care Orders: Significant Harm)* [2000], a nurse was interviewed under caution by the police following a patient's death over alleged drug misuse. The information obtained was insufficient to bring criminal charges, so the police passed the tapes to the nursing regulatory body for them to investigate the nurse's fitness to practise. She claimed a breach of confidence.

   The Court of Appeal held that comments made in police interviews were confidential and remained so even if not used in criminal proceedings. However, disclosure to a regulatory body could be justified in the absence of consent, if it was necessary for the public good to allow the regulatory body to properly investigate the allegations.

Disclosure to protect a third party

The law accepts that there may be circumstances where disclosure of confidential information is necessary in order to protect a third party, particularly where this concerns a vulnerable adult or child. Midwives need to consider all the circumstances and use their professional judgement, informed by reference to the common law, to decide if the public interest in protecting the third party outweighs the public interest in keeping confidential information secret, as shown in the following case study.

CASE STUDY: No breach in protecting children

In *Re L (Care Proceedings: Disclosure to Third Party)* [2000], a paediatric nurse sought an injunction preventing a local authority passing information about her mental health problem to the NMC following care proceedings concerning her and her child. The court allowed the disclosure, holding that the right of the nurse and her child to confidentiality had to be balanced against the public interest in protecting others from a nurse whose fitness to practise had been called into doubt.

Disclosure to prevent or detect a serious crime

There may be circumstances where a midwife is made aware that a woman has committed or intends to commit a crime. Before disclosing such information, it will be necessary for the midwife to weigh the seriousness of the crime against the counter-vailing public interest in maintaining the confidentiality of the woman's health information. The need for a serious crime to have been involved before disclosure is justified in the public interest is highlighted not from a midwifery case but one from mental healthcare (see case study below). As a Court of Appeal case, midwives can use the principles and precedent it establishes to inform their own practice.

CASE STUDY: No breach in preventing a crime

In *W v Egdell* [1990], a doctor was commissioned by W's solicitor to prepare a report for his upcoming appeal against detention under the Mental Health Act 1983. W had been an in-patient at a special hospital for 10 years after he shot five

---

CASE STUDY *continued*

people and was now seeking discharge or relocation to a less secure unit. His consultant psychiatrist supported W's appeal as he felt he had made good progress. However, the doctor's report strongly opposed his relocation and pointed out W's continued interest in firearms and explosives. On receiving the report, W's solicitor withdrew the appeal, which prompted the doctor to send a copy to the medical director of the hospital, as he felt the patient was deceiving his doctors. W then sued for breach of confidence.

The court held that the doctor's duty of confidence to W had to be weighed against the public interests in preventing crime. He was justified in taking this course of action as W posed a real risk to public safety, and the medical team at the hospital were entitled to full information relating to his dangerousness.

It can be seen from this case that midwives would be justified in disclosing information where the crime represents a real risk to public safety – that is, there must be a need to prevent or detect a serious crime to justify breaching a woman's confidentiality, as the countervailing public interest in maintaining sensitive health information would generally outweigh disclosure.

It is very interesting to contrast the disclosure in *W v Egdell* [1990] with the earlier case of *X v Y and Others* [1988], where two doctors in general practice had their HIV status revealed to a national newspaper by employees of a health authority (see page 146). Here, the court held that there was a breach of confidentiality, as there was no public interest to justify overriding the duty of confidence owed to the doctors.

Where a midwife believes he or she is justified in disclosing information about a patient, that disclosure must be to an appropriate source. Indeed, the court in *W v Egdell* [1990] stressed that, while the doctor was right to pass on information to other doctors in Broadmoor about W's dangerousness, he could not lawfully sell the contents of his report to a newspaper. Nor could he, without a breach of the law as well as professional etiquette, discuss the case in a learned article or in his memoirs or in gossiping with friends, unless he took steps to conceal the identity of the patient.

Statutes that modify the duty of confidence

There are three ways in which a statute can modify the duty of confidence owed by a midwife. The statute might:

- reinforce the common law obligation by providing penalties for unjustified disclosure;
- give the midwife the power to disclose information in specific circumstances if he or she considers it appropriate to do so;
- require the midwife to disclose information under specified conditions, leaving him or her with no choice but to pass on the information.

Statutes that reinforce the common law duty of confidence

Information about sexually transmitted infections (STIs) is considered particularly sensitive and private, and you should never assume that women are happy for this information to be shared unless it has a direct and significant bearing on their healthcare. To ensure that confidential information regarding STIs remains private, the general duty of confidence is reinforced by the provisions of the AIDS (Control) Act 1987, the NHS (Venereal Diseases) Regulations 1974, the National Health Service Act 1977 and the National Health Service Trusts and Primary Care Trusts (Sexually Transmitted Diseases) Directions 2000. Under these provisions, every NHS Trust and PCT must take all necessary steps to ensure that any information capable of identifying an individual examined or treated for any STI, including HIV and AIDS, shall not be disclosed except:

- where there is explicit consent to do so;
- for the purpose of communicating that information to a medical practitioner, or to a person employed under the direction of a medical practitioner in connection with the treatment of persons suffering from such disease or the prevention of the spread thereof;
- for the purpose of such treatment or prevention.

Similarly, the provisions of the Human Fertilisation & Embryology Act 1990 and the Human Fertilisation and Embryology (Disclosure of Information) Act 1992 apply restrictions on disclosure to fertilisation and embryo treatment where individuals can be identified. The explicit consent of the person is usually required before disclosure can be authorised, unless it is concerns:

- the provision of treatment services, or any other description of medical, surgical or obstetric services, for the individual giving the consent;
- the carrying out of an audit of clinical practice; or
- the auditing of accounts.

Statutes that empower the health professional to disclose information

The provisions of such statutes give the health professional the power to disclose. It is for the health professional to decide whether in all the circumstances it is appropriate to disclose the information.

Under section 251 of the National Health Service Act 2006, the Secretary of State for Health can make regulations to set aside the common law duty of confidentiality for medical purposes, where it is not possible to use anonymised information and where seeking individual consent is not practicable. For example, the first regulations allowed for the use of information to create and monitor cancer registers and for the surveillance and monitoring of communicable diseases that represent a risk to public health (The Health Service (Control of Patient Information) Regulations (SI 2002/1438) 2002).

Section 251 of the NHS Act 2006 also provides a power to ensure that identifiable information that is required to support a range of work, such as clinical audit, record validation and research, can be used without consent.

Other examples include:

- the Crime and Disorder Act 1998, section 115, which allows for disclosure of information to the police, local authorities or health authorities, where the disclosure is necessary or expedient for the purposes of that Act, such as, for example, the prevention of crime or disorder;
- the Anti-Terrorism, Crime and Security Act 2001, section 17, which allows disclosure to be made for fairly broad purposes relating to criminal investigation and prosecution.

Statutes that require information to be disclosed under specific circumstances

Under these statutory provisions health professionals, such as midwives, have no discretion over whether or not to disclose the information. They are obliged to do so by law, as illustrated in the following case study.

CASE STUDY: Disclosure under the Road Traffic Act 1988

Under the provisions of the Road Traffic Act 1988, there is a duty to disclose information relating to road traffic offences when asked to do so. In *Hunter v Mann* [1974], a doctor was successfully prosecuted for refusing to disclose information that would have revealed the identity of a person driving dangerously. He had refused on the grounds that it had been acquired solely through the relationship of doctor and patient, and to divulge it would be a breach of his professional duty of confidence. The court held that the doctor had been rightly convicted, as the duty imposed by road traffic laws to give information that may lead to the identification of the driver of a vehicle overrides a health professional's duty of confidence to the patient.

Other statutes that require disclosure of information under specific circumstances include:

- the Public Health (Control of Disease) Act 1984 and its regulations, which require a doctor to notify the local authority of the particulars of any person who is suffering from a notifiable disease or food poisoning;
- the National Health Service (Notification of Births) Regulations 1982 (SI 1982/286), which require any person attending a mother to notify the district medical officer of the birth of a child born dead or alive after the twenty-eighth week of pregnancy.
- the Misuse of Drugs (Notification of Supply to Addicts) Regulations 1973, which require a doctor to notify the Home Office of any person he or she considers, or has reasonable grounds to suspect of being, addicted to a notifiable drug.

Disclosing anonymised information

Information is provided by women in confidence and must be treated as such, so long as it remains capable of identifying the woman it relates to. However, anonymised information is not considered confidential and may be used with few constraints. Information that does not identify an individual directly, and that cannot reasonably be used to determine identity, is considered to be anonymous information.

Effective anonymisation requires more than just the removal of names and addresses. A full postcode, an NHS number, or even the name of the ward with the date of admission to hospital, can be strong identifiers, along with other information such as a date of birth, particularly if looked at in combination with other data items.

Anonymised patient information can be used for a range of purposes, such as audit, effective planning of services, research, education and even inclusion in assignments and journal articles.

Disclosing information with appropriate care

The general duty of confidence imposed on registered midwives requires that patient information is kept confidential and must not be disclosed. However, this duty is not absolute and there will be occasions where confidential information will need to be disclosed.

Given that registered midwives will face sanctions from their employer, professional regulatory body and the law for an unwarranted breach of confidence, it is essential that any disclosure of information is done appropriately within the requirements of the duty owed to the patient.

Where you are unclear as to whether a disclosure of information is justified, you should seek advice from a senior colleague or manager. You must also follow the policies on the use and disclosure of patient information that all NHS establishments are required to have, along with the advice given in *Confidentiality: NHS code of practice* (DH, 2003a).

Midwives are required by their rules to discuss the care of mothers with their supervisors. Midwives should ensure that they inform the mothers in their care that any information given will be discussed with their supervisors. The supervisor will be under the same duty of confidence as the midwife. In addition, you must consider the requirements of the NMC's *Code* (2008a) and the law on confidence.

Where a woman has been told that information will be recorded and used for the purpose of delivering effective healthcare, you may share information with other members of the clinical team caring for that individual. Disclosure must be restricted to the clinical team only.

Your duty of confidence generally requires that disclosure of information for purposes other than care and treatment must only be done with explicit consent, unless an exception to that duty applies or the information can be disclosed in an anonymised form (NMC, 2008a) (see above).

Where you intend to disclose confidential information without the explicit consent of the patient, you will need to consider carefully whether an exception to the general duty of confidence applies.

Caldicott Guardians

Each NHS organisation has a guardian of person-based clinical information who oversees the arrangements for the use and sharing of that information. Caldicott Guardians ensure that person-identifiable information is only shared for justified purposes and that only the minimum necessary information is shared in each case.

Every use or flow of identifiable information must be regularly justified and routinely tested against the principles developed in the Caldicott Report, which require NHS organisations to:

- justify the purpose(s) for using confidential information;
- only use it when absolutely necessary;
- use the minimum that is required;
- ensure that access is on a strict need-to-know basis;
- ensure that everyone understands his or her responsibilities;
- understand and comply with the law.

Caldicott Guardians play a key role in ensuring that the NHS satisfies the highest practical standards for handling person-identifiable information. They will actively support work to facilitate and enable information sharing and advise on options for the lawful and ethical processing of information to ensure appropriate information sharing.

C H A P T E R   S U M M A R Y

- Maintaining the confidentiality of a woman's health information is a fundamental element of professional conduct and ethical practice for all registered midwives.
- Women pass on sensitive information in confidence and expect you to respect their privacy by ensuring the confidentiality of the information they give.
- A duty of confidence is imposed on midwives to reassure women that their health information will be respected. The duty is imposed by all contracts of employment in the NHS, the NMC's *Code* and the law.
- The duty of confidence imposed on midwives is not absolute and is subject to a range of exceptions that justify disclosure.
- Consent from the woman allowing disclosure of confidential information is the starting presumption in law. Consent to disclose confidential information with other members of the clinical team may be implied where the woman has been informed.
- Where a woman refuses to allow information to be disclosed to other health professionals involved in her care, it could result in limited care and treatment.
- There are a number of exceptions allowing disclosure to appropriate sources without consent. The public interest exception covers a broad range of situations that allow for confidential information to be disclosed without consent.
- A statute can modify the duty of confidence owed by a midwife.
- Anonymised information is not considered confidential and may be used with few constraints.
- It is essential that any disclosure of information is done appropriately within the requirements of the duty of confidence.
- Each NHS organisation has a guardian of person-based clinical information, known as a Caldicott Guardian, who oversees the arrangements for the use and sharing of clinical information.

Knowledge review

Having completed the chapter, how would you now rate your knowledge of the following topics?

	Good	Adequate	Poor
1. Your duty of confidence to women in your care.			
2. The exceptions to the general duty of confidence.			
3. How to disclose patient information appropriately.			

Where you're not confident in your knowledge of a topic, what will you do next?

Further reading

A recommended read for general guidance on the role and application of the duty of confidence in the NHS is provided by:

Department of Health (DH) (2003) *Confidentiality: NHS code of practice.* London: DH.

For an insight into service users' views on the need for confidentiality and information sharing, we recommend:

NHS Information Authority (NHSIA) (2002) *Share with Care!: People's views on consent and confidentiality of patient information.* London: NHSIA.

Useful websites

www.connectingforhealth.nhs.uk NHS Connecting for Health, which supports the NHS in providing better, safer care, by delivering computer systems and services that improve how information is stored and accessed. It has a range of sources on confidentiality.

www.dh.gov.uk/en/Managingyourorganisation/Informationpolicy/Patientconfidentialit yandcaldicottguardians/index.htm Department of Health website that provides information on confidentiality and health records.

Chapter 10

Negligence

NMC Standards for Pre-registration Midwifery Education

This chapter will address the following competencies:

Domain: Professional and ethical practice

- Practise in accordance with The Code: Standards of conduct, performance and ethics for nurses and midwives (NMC, 2008a), within the limitations of the individual's own competence, knowledge and sphere of professional practice, consistent with the legislation relating to midwifery practice.
- Practise in accordance with relevant legislation. This will include:
  - practising within the contemporary legal framework of midwifery;
  - managing the complexities arising from ethical and legal dilemmas.

Chapter aims

After reading this chapter, you will be able to:

- explain the tort of negligence;
- describe the elements of a negligence action;
- outline the extent of a midwife's duty of care;
- understand how the standard of midwifery care is established by law;
- identify situations where carelessness becomes a crime.

Introduction

This chapter considers how the law imposes a minimum standard on the care you provide to women through the law of negligence. At the beginning of the chapter the financial cost of negligence to the NHS is introduced and the legal obligation to act carefully when providing care and treatment to childbearing women is stressed. This is followed by what constitutes the tort of negligence in healthcare. The extent of your duty as a midwife and how the law determines the standard of care required are discussed. The chapter concludes with a discussion of negligence as a criminal act and the likely consequences if your carelessness results in the death of a woman or her baby.

In the course of their duties it is possible for midwives to make careless mistakes that harm women in their care. Although such mistakes might not be intentional, the resulting harm can nevertheless have a profound effect on the lives of the women and their babies. In order to minimise and discourage such carelessness and provide a remedy for those harmed by the mistakes of others, the law imposes a standard of care on midwives. Therefore, where a midwife's failure to meet this standard results in harm to a woman or her child, he or she will be held to account for carelessness through the law of negligence.

The number of NHS negligence claims has been rising steadily over recent years. In 2008–09, the NHS Litigation Authority received 6,080 claims of clinical negligence and 3,743 claims of non-clinical negligence against NHS bodies. About £769 million was paid out in connection with clinical negligence claims, including £226 million for maternity claims (NHSLA, 2009).

Facing a negligence action is a daunting prospect. Apart from any damages that may be awarded to the person harmed, the midwife concerned faces having his or her professional integrity and good name challenged in court and may face further action being taken against them by their employer and regulatory body.

What is negligence?

Where a midwife acts in a careless way and causes an injury to a mother or baby, that midwife will be liable in negligence for any resulting harm.

The standard generally imposed by law is based on the hypothetical 'reasonable man [sic]'. Negligence can be defined as an omission to do something a reasonable man would do, or to do something a prudent and reasonable man would not do (*Blyth v Birmingham Waterworks* (1856)). For professionals such as midwives, that test extends to what a reasonable body of their peers would have done in the same circumstances, as illustrated below.

CASE STUDY: Was the midwife careless?

In *Lobb v Hartlepool & East Durham NHS Trust* [2001], a child sued a midwife who she claimed had fallen below the standard expected of her. The child argued that, because of the midwife's carelessness, she suffered an injury at birth to her brachial plexus.

The court, however, disagreed, holding that throughout the labour the midwife had exercised her clinical judgement in accordance with the practice of a respected body of midwives and was not careless. She was therefore not liable in negligence.

A woman who suffers harm as a result of a midwife's carelessness can claim for damages. Negligence is, therefore, a form of actionable harm and, if your act or omission causes harm, you could be liable. Where no harm occurs as a result of carelessness, the woman cannot bring an action against the midwife.

The tort of negligence has been developed in English law under the common law provisions. These are a series of judicial decisions and precedents that have the authority of tests to be satisfied if a case is to be successful. The word 'tort' is derived from Norman French meaning 'wrong, mischief, injury, or calamity', and from Latin 'tortus' meaning twisted. Tort is now defined as a civil wrong.

To establish negligence in law, three conditions must be met:

- the person who is considered at fault for the negligence, such as the midwife, must owe the person who has suffered the harm, the woman or baby, a duty of care;
- that duty of care must have been breached, which means that the standard of care given by the midwife must fall below that expected by law;
- as a result of that breach in the standard of care, harm was caused to the person.

Duty of care

In a case of negligence the first element that must be established is whether there is a duty of care owed to the individual concerned. The tort of negligence does not impose a general duty to act carefully on everyone. Instead it lays down standards for particular circumstances and, if someone fails to reach those standards and damage is caused, that is negligence. These are called duty situations and the nature of the relationship gives rise to a duty of care. This duty has also been described by the courts as a duty to take care or a duty to be careful (*Bolitho v City & Hackney HA* [1998]). Therefore, there is a legal obligation to ensure that your acts or omissions do not cause harm to the person to whom you owe that duty.

When deciding if a duty of care arises, the courts rely on previous cases, known as precedent, to guide them. The relationship between midwives and the women in their care is a duty situation and gives rise to a duty of care (*Kent v Griffiths & Others* [2000]).

Where novel situations arise and there are no previous cases to follow, the court uses a three-stage test to decide whether a duty arises.

1. It was reasonably foreseeable that someone would be harmed by a careless act or omission.
   - The test is based on the reasonable foreseeability of harm – that is, would a reasonable person have foreseen that harm would have been caused by the act or omission in question?
2. It is shown that there is a relationship (legal proximity) between the parties.
   - In *Donoghue v Stevenson* [1932], the court established the neighbour principle for determining proximity. The court found that you owe a duty to those who in law are your neighbours – that is, persons who are so closely and directly affected by your act or omission that you ought reasonably to have them in contemplation as being so affected when directing your mind to the acts or omissions in question.
3. It is just and reasonable to impose a duty of care in these circumstances.
   - There are some circumstances where the courts believe that imposing a duty is not just and reasonable and so no duty of care arises. For example, in *JD v East Berkshire Community Health NHS Trust* [2003], parents who had unfounded allegations of child abuse made against them sued the Trust for damages due to psychiatric harm. The court held that it was not just and reasonable to impose a duty in these circumstances, as the paramount concern was the child, and if a midwife had suspicions he or she must be able to report it without having to worry about being sued by parents.

All of these elements were drawn together by the court in the novel circumstances detailed in the following case study.

CASE STUDY: The late-running ambulance

In *Kent v Griffiths and Others* [2000], a pregnant woman suffering recurring severe asthma attacks at home summoned her doctor, who dialled 999 for an ambulance. The dispatcher assured the doctor that an ambulance would be sent immediately, but it took some 40 minutes to arrive. The ambulance should have arrived within 14 minutes, and the crew falsified its response time in their logbook. The woman suffered a respiratory arrest and was brain damaged, and her baby miscarried. She sued the ambulance service for personal injury.

The ambulance service argued that they did not owe the patient a duty of care as they were an emergency service who provided a service to the public, not to individual patients.

The court held that the ambulance service was part of the health service and owed a duty of care to the woman as:

- it was reasonably foreseeable that harm would be caused if they acted in a careless way;
- they knew the name and address of the patient so had a legal proximity in the same way as other health professionals;
- it was just and reasonable to impose a duty of care on the ambulance service towards the woman.

Taking so long, without reasonable excuse, to arrive was careless and a breach of the duty of care.

Activity 10.1   *Critical thinking*

While on duty on the maternity ward, you accidentally spill some water in the main corridor. The wet floor is not clearly visible and can be a potential hazard for those using the corridor.

- Who will you owe a duty of care to in this situation? Answer this question by focusing on the neighbour principle.

An outline answer is given at the end of the chapter.

The scope of the duty of care

The extent of the duty of care owed by a healthcare professional is very wide and covers every facet of your involvement with those in your care. Lord Diplock, in *Sidaway v Bethlem Royal Hospital* [1985], described it as:

> *a single comprehensive duty covering all the ways in which [a midwife] is called on to exercise their skill and judgement in the improvement of the physical and mental condition of the patient.*

Therefore, the scope of your duty of care as a midwife includes:

- the care given;
- giving advice;
- explaining to patients the risks inherent in a procedure;

- the standard of your handwriting when giving instructions, or writing a prescription or a report;
- the standard of your record keeping in terms of legibility, clarity and content;
- the timing of a decision to act;
- seeking assistance from others;
- failing to seek assistance when undertaking a task;
- failing to recognise the limits of your competence;
- failing to report sub-standard care.

Duty of care and psychiatric harm

Psychiatric harm occurs in law where a victim suffers a mental disorder as the result of another's carelessness. Nervous shock was the quaint term used to describe this psychiatric harm. As its name suggests, the harm must occur as a result of a sudden mental shock caused by circumstances that were so exceptional they horrified the victim (*Ward v Leeds Teaching Hospitals NHS Trust* [2004]).

CASE STUDY: *The fainting barmaid*

In *Delieu v White & Sons* [1901], a pregnant barmaid feared for her life after a dray horse crashed through the bar where she worked. She claimed she had suffered psychiatric harm as a result and prematurely gave birth soon after. In awarding damages, the judge agreed that the barmaid had suffered a shock as she was in reasonable fear of immediate personal injury to herself.

The difficulty with cases of psychiatric harm for the courts is the determination of foreseeability of harm and the credibility of evidence of a mental disorder, which is not as easy to see as a broken leg or cut face. The courts therefore restrict the duty of care on the potential victims of a careless action, depending on whether the person is a primary or secondary victim.

Primary and secondary victims

Primary victims are those who are directly involved in the incident. Primary victims of psychiatric harm are treated by the court in the same way as a person who suffers a physical injury due to another's carelessness, as in the case study that follows.

CASE STUDY: *Witnesses to a traumatic birth*

In *Tredegett & Tredegett v Bexley HA* [1994], parents witnessed the negligent birth of their child, who died some 48 hours later. The court found that they were primary victims because of the degree of involvement in the birth and were both entitled to recover damages for the shocking events that they had witnessed and that had left them with pathological grief disorder.

Secondary victims are those who are not directly involved in a negligent incident but are witnesses or bystanders. In these cases, the courts impose restrictions on the way a duty of care arises. The victim must:

- not be abnormally susceptible to psychiatric illness;
- have suffered psychiatric harm that occurred through shock;

- be in physical proximity to the accident or its aftermath;
- have had a close personal or familial relationship with the accident victim.

CASE STUDY: *Mother wrongly told of baby's death*

In *Allin v City & Hackney HA* [1996], a mother suffered shock and post-traumatic stress disorder when she was told that her newborn baby had died, only to discover some hours later that the child was in fact alive. The court found that the mother was a secondary victim and it was foreseeable that such news would be likely to cause psychiatric harm.

Breach in the duty of care

Once it is established that a duty of care is owed, the second question is whether that duty was breached – that is, did the standard of care fall below that required by law?

CASE STUDY: *Failure to warn of baby's disability*

In *Rand v East Dorset HA* [2000], an woman was not told that a test showed her unborn child had Down's syndrome. She suffered shock and depression at seeing her child when born, and on discovering its disability, and recovered damages for negligence.

   The court held that failing to warn the mother about her child's disability fell below the standard required of a midwife, and consequently liability in negligence arose.

Where the person considered to be at fault for a negligent act or omission is a professional, skilled person, such as a midwife, the law modifies the 'reasonable man' test to take account of the skill involved. In *Bolam v Friern HMC* [1957], the court established that:

[t]he test is that of the ordinary skilled person exercising and professing to have that special skill. A professional need not possess the highest expert skill as it is well established in law that it is sufficient if they exercise the ordinary skill of an ordinary competent professional exercising that particular skill or art.

The test is well established in healthcare law and is known as the *Bolam* test. In *Bolitho v City & Hackney HA* [1998], the House of Lords described the *Bolam* test as the *locus classicus* (the traditional basis) of the test for the standard of care required of a doctor or any other person professing some skill or competence. The standard of care is therefore determined by what a responsible body of professional opinion would have done in the same situation. In midwifery, the standard of care will be determined by what a responsible body of midwives would have done in the same situation.

   This approach allows for different schools of thought within a profession. As long as the practice conforms to a standard accepted by a responsible body of opinion, it meets the standard required in law. If not, as the following case study shows, the midwife will be liable in negligence.

CASE STUDY: Midwife exercising clinical judgement

In *Wisniewski v Central Manchester HA* [1998], a midwife appealed against a finding of negligence in relation to the management of a labour where a child suffered cerebral palsy. The child argued that the midwife's failure to call a doctor, who would have performed a caesarean, had caused the disability. The Court of Appeal found the finding of negligence to be correct, as no reasonable midwife would have managed the birth in that way. In their view, she was overconfident in her own abilities to make clinical judgements for which she was not qualified and this had resulted in avoidable harm to the baby.

The law requires a person professing to have a particular skill or art to exercise to the standard of the ordinary professional skilled to that level. Two important qualifications emerge from this principle.

First, the more a professional puts themselves forward as an expert, the higher the standard expected of them. It is the post not the person that carries the duty. The law expects a higher standard of care from the senior midwife than from her junior colleagues. A case arising from the care of a neonate illustrates this first qualification.

CASE STUDY: Higher standard bestowed on experts

In *Wilsher v Essex HA* [1988], a junior doctor needed to take arterial blood gas from a neonate but was unsure if the cannula was in an artery. He asked a specialist registrar, a relatively senior doctor, to check his work and he confirmed that it was in an artery. Regrettably, the cannula was in a vein and a false reading was given, resulting in the neonate being given too much oxygen, causing eye damage.

The House of Lords found that, as the specialist registrar was putting himself forward as an expert, the junior doctor had discharged his duty of care on to the expert, who was negligent in not realising that the sample was venous not arterial blood.

Similarly, when a student midwife asks a more senior colleague to check their intervention with a woman or her baby, the duty of care is discharged on to that colleague, who would be liable if harm resulted from carelessness.

Second, the requirement to perform to the standard of the ordinary person exercising that skill means that there is a minimum level of competence below which no person can fall. Inexperience is therefore no defence to an allegation of negligence. If you profess to have a particular skill, you must perform to the standard of the ordinary midwife. This is best illustrated by a case concerning a familiar skill, driving a car.

CASE STUDY: Liability of the learner driver

In *Nettleship v Weston* [1971], a learner driver was given lessons by an instructor, who made sure the car was properly insured. Weston was a careful learner, but on the third lesson she failed to straighten out after turning left, and struck a lamp standard, breaking Nettleship's kneecap.

> ## CASE STUDY *continued*
>
> The court held that a learner driver owes a duty to their instructor to drive with proper skill and care, the test being that of the ordinary careful driver. It was no defence to say that he or she was a learner doing their best. The duty of care owed by a learner driver was the same as that owed by every driver, and Weston was liable for damages.

When the principles in this case are applied to midwifery, it can be seen that a minimum level of competence is expected even of student midwives if they are caring for women and babies. This is the standard of the ordinary midwife. It is important, therefore, to acknowledge the limitations in your practice and seek more senior assistance, so that you do not carelessly cause harm by practising beyond your competence. This will ensure that you benefit from the help and advice of the colleague. It will also demonstrate that you have discharged your duty of care towards the woman.

> ## Activity 10.2   *Reflection*
>
> What action would you take if you were unsure how to carry out an intervention on a woman in your care?
>
> *An outline answer is given at the end of the chapter.*

Emergencies

One exception to the principle that a midwife will be judged according to the standard of a reasonably experienced midwife is provided where emergency treatment is required.

Where treatment decisions are taken in an emergency, a midwife will not be found negligent simply because a reasonably competent midwife would have made a different decision given more time and information.

There is no negligence when a health professional makes an immediate decision whether to treat, when the treatment was subsequently found to have been unnecessary (*Wilson v Swanson* (1956)). Furthermore, the standard of skill required in providing treatment may in itself be lower. As Lord Justice Mustill commented in *Wilsher v Essex HA* [1988]:

> An emergency may overburden the available resources, and, if an individual is forced by circumstances to do too many things at once, the fact that he does one of them incorrectly should not lightly be taken as negligence.

The role of the courts in determining the standard of care

Generally, the courts are content to allow the profession to set the standard of care for a particular treatment or intervention. The essence of the *Bolam* test is that midwives act in accordance with a practice accepted by a responsible body of professional opinion.

However, the court is the final arbiter of the professional standard of care and, although it must accept that there are different schools of thought about how to best provide treatment within a profession, it can reject a standard where it does not consider that the standard stands up to logical analysis (*Bolitho v City & Hackney HA* [1998]).

Activity 10.3   *Critical thinking*

In *Hucks v Cole* (1968), a woman was expecting her third child when she noticed a septic spot on her finger. She gave birth three days later in hospital. The following day, a nurse noticed the spot and another one on her toe. The doctor prescribed a five-day course of tetracycline and sent a swab to pathology.

The pathologist's report stated that the bacteria were resistant to tetracycline, but the doctor decided to stick to the five-day course he had prescribed.

Hucks was discharged at the end of the five days despite the septic spots not having healed. She soon became seriously ill with fulminating septicaemia.

At the trial, evidence was given by other doctors that they would not have changed the prescribed treatment.

- Do you think the doctor's actions stand up to logical analysis?

Please do not move on to the next part until you are ready for the answer.

In this case, the judge held that (despite the evidence of the doctors) no reasonable doctor would allow a patient to continue with a course of treatment when they knew it to be ineffective. The standard of care suggested by the doctors did not stand up to logical analysis and would be rejected. This was later approved by the House of Lords in *Bolitho v City & Hackney HA* [1998], when they held that:

> [Where], in a rare case, it can be demonstrated that the professional opinion is not capable of withstanding logical analysis, the judge is entitled to hold that the body of opinion is not reasonable or responsible.
>
> (Lord Browne-Wilkinson at 240)

Therefore, it is important that midwives base their practice on sound evidence and research. You will not be exonerated because others are also negligent or common professional practice is slack (*Reynolds v North Tyneside HA* [2002]). You must keep your practice up to date and informed by reference to improvements and amendments introduced through changes in the law.

Guidance on best practice

NHS organisations have policies and procedures to inform best practice so as to improve care standards. These are supplemented by guidance from bodies such as the National Institute for Health and Clinical Excellence (NICE), professional organisations such as the Royal College of Midwives (RCM) and the NMC, and strategies such as the National Service Frameworks (NSFs). Midwives are able to use these to inform their practice. For example, an obstetrics senior registrar performed an instrumental delivery at a time when guidance from the Royal College of Gynaecologists and Obstetricians stipulated that it was not acceptable medical practice to do. The child sustained injuries at birth and the registrar was found to be negligent. The court held that these guidelines, which would have been circulated to medical staff prior to the date of the incident, gave clear authoritative indication that to attempt instrumental delivery at that time (prior to full dilation of the cervix) was not acceptable practice (*DF (by her litigation friend and mother CF) v St George's Healthcare NHS Trust* [2005]).

CASE STUDY: Hospital policy and research evidence

In *Reynolds v North Tyneside HA* [2002], a woman who was admitted in labour was not given a vaginal examination for six hours, at which point a prolapsed cord was discovered and an emergency caesarean carried out. The child suffered cerebral palsy and sued. The hospital argued that its policy did not require the immediate vaginal examination of the woman; however, the pre-eminent text book of the day suggested that such an examination was necessary where a woman was in labour.

The court held that the hospital policy was not based on sound research evidence and did not stand up to logical analysis, and there had been a breach in the standard of care, causing harm to the child. The hospital was therefore negligent.

Causation

Once it is established that the standard of care required in law has been breached due to the carelessness of the midwife, it is then necessary to consider what effect this has had on the woman and her baby. This stage is known as 'causation' or the 'causal link', where it must be established that the breach in the standard of care caused the harm.

It is generally for the person who has suffered the wrong (the claimant) to prove causation. The claimant must prove on the balance of probabilities that care fell below the standard of a reasonably competent person and caused the harm. There is a distinction between causation in fact and causation in law.

Causation in fact is based on the 'but for' test – that is, but for your carelessness the patient would not have suffered harm.

CASE STUDY: Application of the 'but for' test

In *Jones v North West SHA* [2010], a baby suffered cerebral palsy as a result of shoulder dystocia, which delayed the delivery and compressed the cord, causing anoxia. The baby's mother contended that she had not been told of the risk of this happening, and if she had been told she would have elected to have a caesarean section.

The court found that the midwife should have told the baby's mother of the risk of shoulder dystocia, but that this oversight was not the cause of the cerebral palsy, because, even if she had been told, the woman's religious beliefs meant that she would have been unlikely to agree to a caesarean section.

Causation in law requires the court to determine whether the defendant is liable as a matter of law. This is determined by the principle that the defendant will not be held liable in law if the damage is too remote from the original negligent act.

CASE STUDY: Damages for an unborn child

In *Watt v Rama* [1972], a baby suffered serious injuries as a result of the negligent driving of the defendant. At the time of the accident, the plaintiff was *en ventre sa mere* (in the womb or unborn) and the action was brought on her behalf after birth. The driver argued that liability for the harm to a child not born at the time of the accident was too remote.

The court found that injury to a pregnant woman was foreseeable and, where the injury does not arise contemporaneously with the negligence, the duty of care crystallises when the baby is born alive. The harm suffered by the baby was therefore not too remote.

Res ipsa loquitur

While it is generally for the complainant to prove that a breach in the standard of care caused them harm, there is a principle that allows the burden of proof to shift in certain circumstances.

The principle of *res ipsa loquitur*, or 'the thing speaks for itself', applies when three key conditions apply:

- there is no explanation for the accident;
- harm does not normally happen if care is taken;
- the instrument causing the accident is in the defendant's control.

The principle requires the respondent to show that he or she did not act negligently, by shifting the burden of proof from the complainant to the respondent. An example of *res ipsa loquitur* can be seen in the next case study.

CASE STUDY: Contaminated epidural anaesthesia

In *Sutcliffe v Aintree Hospitals NHS Trust* [2008], after giving birth with the aid of an epidural a woman developed inflammation of tissues within the spine, with severe neurological and physical consequences. The court found that the inflammation was caused by contamination of the spinal anaesthetic with a cleansing agent, chlorhexidine, at some stage during the anaesthetic procedure. *Res ipsa loquitur* applied as this could only have happened if there had been a breach of duty on the part of one or other of the two clinicians involved in the procedure.

Negligence as a crime

Negligence is generally associated with the civil law. It is the law's way of imposing a standard of care on professionals such as midwives, and it provides redress by way of compensation for those harmed by another's careless act or omission.

In cases where the negligent act of a healthcare professional, such as a midwife, causes the death of a person in their care, a crime may have been committed and a charge of gross negligence manslaughter may be brought against the midwife. In *R v Bateman* [1925], the court decided that gross negligence occurs when someone shows such disregard for the life and safety of other persons as to constitute a crime worthy of punishment. In healthcare, the issue of gross negligence arose in *R v Misra & Srivastava* [2004], where two doctors were found guilty of gross negligence when they failed to heed the warnings of nurses that a patient was seriously ill. The patient subsequently died of toxic shock. The judge held that:

> [a] health professional would be told that grossly negligent treatment which exposed a patient to the risk of death, and caused it, would constitute manslaughter.

This was the case in *R v Adomako* [1995], where the defendant, an anaesthetist, failed to notice for four minutes that an endotracheal tube had become disconnected during an operation. Although an alarm sounded, the tube was not checked until the patient suffered a cardiac arrest. An expert witness for the prosecution stated that a competent anaesthetist should have spotted the problem within 15 seconds. The House of Lords held that gross negligence would apply where a patient's death occurs as the result of a health professional:

- displaying an indifference to an obvious risk of injury to the patient;
- being aware of the risk of injury to the patient but deciding to run the risk;
- attempting to avoid a known risk in a manner that is so grossly negligent it deserves to be punished;
- displaying inattention or a failure to avert a severe risk.

Based on these tests, a midwife could be convicted of manslaughter if the act or omission exposed the patient to the risk of death and subsequently caused the patient's death.

Where a midwife is found guilty of such an offence, a custodial sentence is likely.

CASE STUDY: *Unlawful killing through gross negligence*

In 2010, an inquest returned a verdict of unlawful killing through gross negligence following the death of a mother two hours after giving birth. A midwife mistakenly gave the mother a strong epidural, Bupivacain, via an intravenous drip. The mother died of a heart attack. The coroner's jury heard that the drug was not stored safely away from intravenous drugs and the midwife failed to check the drugs despite having six opportunities to do so (De Bruxelles, 2010).

As well as individual practitioners facing criminal charges, it is now likely that the midwife's employing organisation would also face charges under the provisions of the Corporate Manslaughter and Corporate Homicide Act 2007. Companies and organisations can be found guilty of corporate manslaughter as a result of serious management failures resulting in a gross breach of a duty of care.

Accountability

As we saw in Chapter 3, registered midwives are not only accountable to the women and babies in their care, but are also accountable to their employer through their contracts and to the NMC through the Nursing and Midwifery Order 2001. Even if it is shown that carelessness did not cause harm, a midwife is likely to face investigation by his or her employer and the NMC.

Under contract law, employers must pay any damages for liability in negligence through the principle of 'vicarious liability'. Employers are liable for the negligent acts or omissions of their employees in the course of their employment. The liability arises whether or not such acts or omissions were specifically authorised by the employer.

In return for this protection, employers expect their employees to carry out their duties with due care and skill. They can hold midwives to account through reasonable disciplinary measures that could include dismissal if an investigation reveals misconduct.

The NHS indemnity scheme covers NHS organisations and their employees, including midwives, and will pay compensation for clinical negligence. Independent midwives do not have the benefit of the NHS indemnity scheme. Since 2005, no commercial insurer has been willing to provide indemnity insurance to cover independent midwives because of the high quantum (compensation) that is often awarded to babies harmed by negligence.

CASE STUDY: *Compensation for clinical accident*

A boy received £8 million compensation in a High Court settlement for failures during his birth that left him severely disabled (Brady, 2008). He was deprived of air for 17 minutes after midwives failed to spot signs of distress in foetal monitoring hours before he was born. The Trust accepted that it was at fault. During the mother's labour, an obstetrician was not called to examine an abnormal cardiotocograph (CTG) indicating foetal distress. Midwives continued to try to manage the delivery and, as a result, the boy sustained brain damage at birth due to a period of near total asphyxia.

The size of compensation payments means that independent midwives must work without insurance. They cannot absolve themselves from a negligence action as this would be contrary to the provisions of the Unfair Contract Terms Act 1977. Independent midwives must tell their clients that they are uninsured and would, therefore, not have the funds to pay any compensation that might be awarded should they be sued.

The fairness and viability of this arrangement is a source of continuing debate. Is it fair to a baby harmed by the negligence of an independent midwife to be denied compensation because the midwife is uninsured?

The EU is proposing a directive on safe, high-quality and efficient cross-border healthcare that includes a requirement that all health professionals must have indemnity insurance in order to practise (European Commission, 2007). Despite initially indicating that it would introduce such a law in the UK, effectively ending the right of independent midwives to practise, the government has instead decided to review the law to see if an alternative solution can be found.

Senior lawyers and patient safety campaigners have now accused the Department of Health and the NMC of choosing to protect the interests of professionals over the needs of mothers and babies, who, until the issue is resolved, cannot get compensation for negligent care.

In *The Code* (NMC, 2008a), the NMC only recommends that registered midwives have professional indemnity insurance. It is, as yet, not compulsory.

- Where a midwife acts in a careless way and causes an injury to another person, such as a woman in labour, that careless midwife will be liable in negligence for any resulting harm.
- Negligence is best defined as actionable harm. In order to establish negligence in law, three conditions must be met: the midwife must owe the woman a duty of care; that duty of care must be breached; and as a result harm was caused to the woman or her baby.
- The relationship between a midwife and a pregnant or labouring woman is one that gives rise to a duty of care. This duty covers all the ways in which a midwife is called on to exercise skill and judgement in the improvement of the physical and mental condition of the patient.
- As a skilled professional, you are expected to carry out your duties to the standard of the ordinary skilled person exercising and professing to have that special skill. The standard of care is determined by what a responsible body of professional opinion would have done in the same situation. The more a midwife puts him- or herself forward as an expert, the higher the standard expected.
- Inexperience is no defence to an allegation of negligence.
- The court can reject a professional standard where it does not consider that the standard stands up to logical analysis.
- The principle of res ipsa loquitur applies when there is no explanation for the accident, harm does not normally happen if care is taken, and the instrument causing the accident is in the defendant's control.
- Grossly negligent treatment that exposes a woman or baby to the risk of death, and causes it, constitutes manslaughter.
- It is essential that midwives carry indemnity insurance to cover them for any damages for which they are personally liable.

Activities: brief outline answers

Activity 10.1: Critical thinking (page 161)

The courts have held that, in law, you owe a duty of care to your neighbour. The court describes 'neighbours' as:

> persons who are so closely and directly affected by your act or omission that you ought reasonably to have them in contemplation as being so affected when directing your mind to the acts or omission in question.

In the case of an accidental spill, you would therefore owe a duty to individuals walking along that corridor because it is reasonably foreseeable that they could be harmed if they slipped on the wet floor.

Activity 10.2: Reflection (page 165)

Given the decision in the case of *Wilsher v Essex HA* [1988], you would be well advised to seek the supervision of a more senior colleague. Should harm occur after consultation with the senior colleague, it will be that professional who will be held liable for negligence, as they have put themselves forward as an expert and a higher standard of care would be expected of them

Knowledge review

Having completed the chapter, how would you now rate your knowledge of the following topics?

	Good	Adequate	Poor
1. The elements of a negligence action.			
2. The standard of care required of you as a skilled professional.			
3. The circumstances where negligence could become a criminal offence.			

Where you're not confident in your knowledge of a topic, what will you do next?

Further reading

To appreciate the court's approach to the standard imposed by a duty of care, it is well worth reading the House of Lords' opinion in:
Bolitho v City and Hackney HA [1998] AC 232, which can be downloaded at **www.bailii. org/uk/cases/UKHL/1997/46.html**

A very interesting document by the Department of Health, which strives to get health professionals to learn from the mistakes of others, is well worth reading for its case studies and cautionary tales:
Department of Health (DH) (2003) *An Organisation with a Memory*. London: DH.

Useful websites

To keep up to date with negligence cases that affect health professionals, see the following:
www.bailii.org The British and Irish Legal Information Institute.
www.nhsla.com The National Health Service Litigation Authority.

You can also access Law Reports from the following, but they both require you to have an Athens account:
www.lawtel.com (a division of law publisher Sweet and Maxwell)
www.lexisnexis.co.uk

Chapter 11

Safeguarding vulnerable women

NMC Standards for Pre-registration Midwifery Education

This chapter will address the following competencies:

Domain: Effective midwifery practice

- Contribute to enhancing the health and social wellbeing of individuals and their communities.

Domain: Professional and ethical practice

- Support the creation and maintenance of environments that promote the health, safety and wellbeing of women, babies and others. This will include:
  - Promoting health, safety and security in the environment in which the midwife is working, whether it be at a woman's home, in the community, a clinic or in a hospital.

Chapter aims

After reading this chapter, you will be able to:

- define the term 'vulnerable adult woman';
- explain the role of the midwife in the safeguarding of vulnerable women and victims of domestic abuse;
- outline the legal remedies available for the safeguarding of vulnerable women and victims of domestic abuse;
- describe how women are protected from abuse by midwives.

Introduction

This chapter considers how the law can be employed by health and social care professionals to protect vulnerable women from abuse. We begin with an agreed definition of a vulnerable adult and then consider what is meant by abuse and the forms it may take. We then summarise the powers available to health and social care authorities to protect the vulnerable from harm, and consider the implications of the Sexual Offences Act 2003. The chapter ends by looking at the vetting and barring scheme introduced by the Safeguarding Vulnerable Groups Act 2006, which seeks to ensure that unsuitable people are prevented from working with adults who are vulnerable.

We saw in Chapter 4 that a key principle of human rights law is the duty on state governments to have laws and policies in place that prevent one person violating the human rights of another. Since 2000, the government departments responsible for health and social care in England, Scotland and Wales have issued policy documents, requiring multi-agency working led by local social services departments to: prevent, identify, investigate, respond to and ameliorate the abuse of vulnerable adults in all settings and to take appropriate action against perpetrators of abuse.

The Department of Health (DH, 2002) issued guidance in its policy document entitled *No Secrets*, in which it defined a vulnerable adult as:

> *a person aged 18 years or over, who is in receipt of or may be in need of community care services by reason of mental or other disability, age or illness and who is or may be unable to take care of him or herself, or unable to protect him or herself against significant harm or exploitation.*

Issued in Wales, a similar document, *In Safe Hands*, reiterated the commitment to promoting independence and safeguarding vulnerable adults (Welsh Assembly Government, 2000).

These documents led to comprehensive adult protection strategies being implemented by social services across the UK to coordinate a process of policy developments for the identification and prevention of abuse of vulnerable adults in all settings. This requires engagement with all sectors, including the sharing of information and the actions necessary to deal with the abusers. Midwives are likely to come into contact with vulnerable adults, either within a community setting or in a hospital setting, when providing a package of care during and after pregnancy. It is essential that all midwives and student midwives are aware of the measures that need to be taken to safeguard women who are vulnerable.

Vulnerable adults

Activity 11.1   *Research and group work*

- Familiarise yourself with the document *No Secrets*, which is available at www.dh.gov.uk/en/Publicationsandstatistics/PublicationsPolicyAndGuidance/DH_4008486. Jot down the main aims of the document.
- In a group assess the strengths and weaknesses of this approach and consider whether it meets the needs of women who are vulnerable.

Please do not move on to the next part until you are ready for the answer.

A number of policy documents have been issued to inform statutory and voluntary agencies that have to deal with people who are vulnerable and that have to safeguard them from abuse. These policies place the responsibility for taking action and investigating complaints with local agencies. In turn, each local authority/NHS Trust has issued its own policy on safeguarding vulnerable adults.

Abuse can be a single act or repeated acts and it may be physical, psychological, verbal, sexual or financial. Essentially, there are two characteristics associated with abuse:

- a vulnerable adult has been hurt or deprived of the care he or she is entitled to;
- the abuse has been meted out by another person or persons.

There are different forms of abuse, as follows.

- **Physical abuse** – including hitting, slapping, overdosage or misuse of medication, undue restraint, or inappropriate sanctions.
- **Sexual abuse** – including rape, sexual assault or sexual acts to which the vulnerable adult has not consented, or could not consent, and/or was pressured into consenting.
- **Psychological abuse** – including threats of harm or abandonment, humiliation, verbal or racial abuse, isolation or withdrawal from services or supportive networks.
- **Financial or material abuse** – including theft, fraud, pressure concerning wills, property or inheritance, and misuse or misappropriation of benefits.
- **Neglect** – including failure to access medical care and services, negligence in the face of risk-taking, failure to give prescribed medication, poor nutrition or lack of heating.

CASE STUDY: Neglect by independent midwife

An uninsured independent midwife was struck off the register for serious professional misconduct as a result of failing to provide an appropriate standard of care.

Her client was left needing reconstructive surgery after the midwife randomly cut her in order to deliver the baby. In the process, the midwife cut the nerves in the arm and neck of the baby, causing Erb's palsy. The midwife failed, among other things, to call for immediate assistance, to have a second midwife present, to document and make relevant observations, such as measurements of fundal heights and foetal heart rates, and failed to recognise that the expected labour might be an obstetric emergency (NMC, 2010a).

The legal framework

There is no specific legislation that deals with vulnerable adult abuse. What we have instead are a number of legislative measures that seek to offer protection. The challenge for midwives rests on their ability to interpret the rights, duties and powers available and apply these to the circumstances in each individual case.

Insofar as midwives are concerned, knowledge of the remedies and powers available is essential in the event that they are confronted with suspected abuse of a vulnerable person. Midwives should have a working knowledge of their organisation's policies concerning the safeguarding of the vulnerable. This enables them to seek appropriate advice from within the organisation about their concerns. It may not be possible to obtain such advice at short notice, in which case a midwife may need to turn to outside agencies such as the police or social services for advice and support. Detecting or recognising abuse is notoriously difficult in practice. A working knowledge of the legal rights of women and clients is helpful in knowing how to address concerns in relation to a vulnerable adult.

Midwives owe negative obligation to the women in their care, in order to ensure that they do not breach their human rights when providing maternity services. Midwives also have a duty to report and take action on allegations of abuse where they know, or ought reasonably to have known, that a woman was being abused (see Chapter 3).

The threshold for state intervention in the case of a vulnerable person is the risk of significant harm, which is defined as:

> [i]ll treatment (including sexual abuse and forms of ill treatment that are not physical); the impairment of, or an avoidable deterioration in, physical or mental health; and the impairment of physical, emotional, social or behavioural development.
>
> (DH, 2002)

In deciding whether any action should be taken, the midwife should uphold the right of a vulnerable woman to make informed choices and to take risks where she is not being unduly intimidated. The available options should be explored with her and her wishes respected, unless these conflict with a statutory duty to intervene, or unless another person or child is considered to be at risk.

The philosophy underpinning this approach is based on the right of service users to make choices and maintain their independence, even if that involves an element of risk. In all circumstances, they should be consulted and involved in decision making as far as possible. Midwives would need to assess the capacity of the individuals involved. The Mental Capacity Act 2005 sets out the general requirements for determining whether a person has capacity and for determining what care and treatment would be in a person's best interests.

CASE STUDY: Best interests of a women with learning disabilities

In Re S (Adult Patient Sterilisation) [2000], an application was made to the court by the mother of a 28-year-old woman who suffered from a severe learning disability, for a declaration that it would be in the woman's best interests to undergo sterilisation. The mother was concerned that her daughter could become pregnant when away from her close supervision. Medical evidence was unanimous in finding that the woman could not give informed consent and that pregnancy would be disastrous for her.

CASE STUDY continued

The court held that the woman's best interests had to consider whether: (a) the treatment was necessary for therapeutic purposes; and (b) there was a less invasive form of treatment available. On balance, the court decided that the woman ought not to undergo the sterilisation operation as it was an irreversible procedure and other reversible options were available, such as the insertion of an intrauterine device.

Where an allegation of abuse is made or there is a serious issue, such as sterilisation or pregnancy, affecting the life of a vulnerable person, the local authority, as the lead agency, is responsible for investigating the matter, setting up a case conference with all interested parties and looking into the available remedies that would safeguard the vulnerable person.

The legal basis for making decisions on behalf of a vulnerable adult is far from straightforward, but there are a number of powers that are available. These include the jurisdiction of the court.

When the court is faced with an application in relation to the welfare of a vulnerable adult, it has to consider what legal authority it is able to act under. Where the issue concerns a person who lacks capacity to make a decision, the Mental Capacity Act 2005 will be the basis of the court's authority (see Chapter 5).

The courts also have an inherent jurisdiction that is wider than the provisions set out in the Mental Capacity Act 2005, as it gives the court authority to take action where a person has capacity but is considered vulnerable and in need of protection. This at first appears odd, given the importance in law of upholding the right of a capable individual to determine for themselves how they should live their lives. It shows that the law recognises that there is a difference between autonomy and capacity. A person may have capacity, but a decision is not an autonomous one where the person is being coerced.

CASE STUDY: *Coercion negatives consent*

In *Re SA (Vulnerable Adult with Capacity: Marriage)* [2005], a woman who had just turned 18 years was at risk of being made the subject of an arranged marriage. She was deaf and unable to speak, and communicated by British sign language. Communication within her family was limited as her parents spoke only Punjabi. She functioned at the intellectual level of a 13 or 14 year old, with a reading age of seven or eight. Expert evidence was that she had capacity to marry as she understood the concept of marriage, including a sexual relationship. However, she would have difficulty in understanding a specific marriage contract to a specific individual involving a change in her country of residence. She did not want to live in Pakistan.

The court found that the woman was to be properly informed, in a manner she could understand, about any specific marriage prior to entering into it. The court exercised a protective jurisdiction in relation to vulnerable adults that was not confined to cases where a vulnerable adult was disabled by mental incapacity from making their own decision or where an adult was unable to communicate their decision. There was a need to intervene to protect this woman from the harm she would suffer if she went through a marriage ceremony with which she did not agree. It was therefore right to exercise the court's protective jurisdiction over her.

In can be seen from the case study that, in the context of the inherent jurisdiction, a vulnerable adult is someone who, whether or not mentally incapacitated, and whether or not suffering from any mental disorder, is unable to take care of themselves or unable to protect themselves against significant harm or exploitation. A vulnerable adult is also someone who is deaf, blind, dumb or substantially handicapped by illness, injury or congenital deformity. This implies that inherent jurisdiction can be used to protect a competent but vulnerable adult from harm or exploitation.

There are now a number of statutes that seek to protect women where the law considers them to be in a vulnerable position.

Forced marriage

The government has acknowledged that midwives, along with other health professionals, are ideally placed to offer early and effective advice and support to women who are the victims of forced marriage (FCO, 2007). It is essential that you are aware of the measures that can be taken to help and protect women who are the victims of forced marriage through the provisions of the Forced Marriage (Civil Protection) Act 2007.

This protection was highlighted in the case of an NHS doctor who was forcibly lured back to Bangladesh and held by her parents until she married a suitor chosen by them. A forced marriage prevention order issued by the UK High Court resulted in the Bangladeshi authorities ordering her release and return to the UK (Green, 2008).

Right to marry

A person can willingly enter into a marriage at 16 years, with parental consent required for those less than 18 years old. However, under section 12c of the Matrimonial Causes Act 1973, a marriage is voidable if *either party to the marriage did not validly consent to it, whether in consequence or duress, mistake, unsoundness of mind or otherwise.*

Arranged marriages and forced marriages

In the first nine months of 2008, over 1,300 incidences of suspected forced marriage involving British citizens and foreign nationals resident in the UK were reported to the Forced Marriage Unit, which is a part of the Foreign & Commonwealth Office (FCO, 2008). In those cases, there were concerns that a person was about to be forced into marriage, or had already been forced to marry. Suspected cases of forced marriage come to the attention of the police, social, health and education services and voluntary organisations.

To properly identify the victim of a forced marriage it is important to differentiate between a forced marriage and an arranged marriage.

- A forced marriage is a marriage in which one or both spouses do not consent to the marriage and duress is involved. Duress can include physical, psychological, financial, sexual or emotional pressure.
- An arranged marriage is a tradition that has operated successfully within many communities and countries for many years. In arranged marriages the families of both spouses take a leading role in arranging the marriage, but the choice whether to accept the arrangement remains with the individuals.

Vulnerable adults with impaired decision-making capacity and who cannot consent to a marriage cannot enter into an arranged marriage. The Mental Capacity Act 2005 states that entering a marriage is a decision that is excluded from the decisions that can be made on behalf of a person who lacks decision-making capacity. In *KC & NNC v City of Westminster & IC* [2008], the Court of Appeal held that the arranged marriage of an autistic man to a woman in Bangladesh, carried out over the telephone, was void as the man lacked capacity to enter into a marriage.

Forced Marriage (Civil Protection) Act 2007

In many situations of forced marriage, the victim may be unable or unwilling to make a complaint. Very often those affected do not want their relatives to be criminalised. The Forced Marriage (Civil Protection) Act 2007 provides a civil remedy to forced marriages. The aim is to give greater protection to victims and potential victims of forced marriage and allow a third party to apply for a forced marriage protection order (FMPO). The provisions give the courts the flexibility to deal sensitively with the circumstances of each individual case and to use remedies that will offer protection to victims without criminalising members of their family.

Forced marriage protection order

Under section 63A(1) of the Family Law Act 1996, a court can make an FMPO for the purposes of protecting a person from being forced into a marriage or to protect a person who has been forced into a marriage. Force includes coercion by threats or other psychological means and includes verbal, psychological and physical force. The forced marriage can be any marriage and can include religious marriages not legally recognised in England and Wales. The conduct that forces a person into marriage does not have to be directed against them. It can be directed against another, including the perpetrator. This covers circumstances where the perpetrator harassed the victim's parents to force the marriage, or the perpetrator threatens suicide if the victim does not submit to marriage.

The court may make an order containing any measures considered appropriate to protect against conduct that may lead to a forced marriage, or to protect a person in a forced marriage. The order may prohibit certain activity or require a person to do something. The court is given a wide discretion to order people to hand over passports or reveal the whereabouts of a person thought to be at risk, and to stop someone from being taken abroad.

Applying for a forced marriage protection order

A person who is to be protected, or a relevant third party, can apply for an FMPO) (Family Law Act 1996, s63C). A relevant third party is someone who can make an application on behalf of a victim of forced marriage. Local authorities can act as relevant third parties, as can local independent domestic violence advisers. A friend, a teacher or the police can also apply with the court's permission.

The court can make an order against a person who is forcing another into entering a marriage. An order can also be made against those who are involved in a forced marriage. Therefore, it will include those who are aiding, abetting, counselling, procuring, encouraging or assisting another person to force another into entering a marriage. An FMPO can be made against a person who is in or outside the UK.

Breaching a forced marriage protection order

Any person who contravenes an FMPO commits an offence and is liable to a fine, a term of imprisonment or both.

The court must attach a power of arrest to any order if the respondent has used or threatened to use violence and there would be no adequate protection without this power of arrest. This allows the police to arrest anyone they suspect of being in breach of the order or a third party who frustrates the terms of the order. For example, if an order were made to prevent a father and mother from forcing their child into a marriage and another family member continued the coercion, the power of arrest could be used against them as well.

Domestic abuse as a midwifery issue

Domestic abuse has replaced domestic violence as the term used to define verbal, sexual, physical, emotional, intimidating or financial abuse that occurs within a family relationship. The Law Commission, in its report on domestic violence and occupation of the family home (Law Commission, 1992), considered domestic violence as too narrow a definition as it described the use or threat of physical force against a victim. However, in the context of the family, abuse extended beyond more typical instances of physical assault to include any form of physical, sexual or psychological molestation or harassment that has a serious detrimental effect upon the health and well-being of the victim, even though there is no violence in terms of assault and battery.

CASE STUDY: Photographs as abuse

In *Johnson v Walton* [1990], a husband was found to be causing molestation to his wife by sending partially nude photographs of her to a national newspaper for publication.

The Chief Medical Officer of England claimed that the effect of domestic violence on the well-being of victims is so great that it represents a major public health issue (DH, 1997b). Midwives are in a unique position to help people who suffer abuse at home. Having contact with women in their own homes puts midwives in a situation where they can identify, assess and respond to domestic abuse. A third of women report their first episode of abuse as occurring during pregnancy and the three key risk factors for domestic abuse are:

- being a woman;
- being pregnant;
- being aged between 16 and 24.

Victims are often reluctant to contact or cooperate with the police or the criminal justice system (CJS) and often suffer as many as 35 episodes of violence before reporting the matter to the police (Bewley et al., 1997). Even where episodes of abuse are reported to the police, victims often later withdraw the complaint and, although the police and Crown Prosecution Service are now encouraged to proceed on the evidence they have compiled (Home Office, 1990), this can prove difficult in practice.

CASE STUDY: Reluctance to proceed with criminal action

In *R v Bigwood* [2000], the court held that the prosecution of a husband for stabbing his wife would not proceed, as the wife had later retracted her complaint, and the use of photographs of her and her home and of a statement compiled from her medical notes amounted to a potential breach of her human rights.

Having contact with a midwife provides an opportunity for early recognition and support of the victim. It also provides an alternative to involving the police and CJS, which victims often wish to avoid.

Asking women about domestic abuse

Victims of domestic abuse are often reluctant to admit that they have suffered domestic abuse, and there are a number or reasons for this.

Concept summary: Some reasons for non-disclosure of domestic violence

- Shame and embarrassment.
- Fear:
    - of an unsympathetic response;
    - of not being believed;
    - of reprisals or escalation of violence from partners;
    - of their children being taken into care;
    - of the police being informed.
- Cultural stigma.
- Lack of awareness that midwives may be able to help.

Taket (2004) suggests that, because of the general reluctance of victims of domestic abuse to come forward and seek help, it is essential that midwives are able to recognise the main signs. Midwives are now encouraged to enquire about domestic abuse as part of a routine antenatal assessment (Salmon et al., 2004). The next concept summary lists the key signs that should trigger a direct enquiry.

Concept summary: Signs of domestic abuse

The Home Office document, *Tackling Domestic Violence: The role of health professionals* (2004), lists the following signs to look out for.

Physical
- Stress-related ailments – headaches, irritable bowel syndrome.
- STIs, vaginal infections or other frequent gynaecological problems.
- Miscarriage or a history of miscarriages.
- Repeated terminations of pregnancy; or stillbirths.
- Premature labour.
- Babies with low birth weight; or fractures to the foetus.
- Forced removal of sutures.
- Bruises on the body, particularly on the breasts and abdomen.
- Injuries to face, head or neck; or multiple injuries in different stages of healing.
- Burns – cigarette burns, rope burns; and hair loss consistent with hair pulling.
- Bilateral injuries; unexplained injuries; or those inconsistent with explanations.
- Unexplained accidents to children.

Concept summary continued

Behavioural

- Frequent A & E visits.
- Appearing fearful, evasive, ashamed, embarrassed.
- Partner answering questions directed to the woman.
- Use of alcohol and drugs (e.g. tranquillisers).
- Eating disorders.
- Frequent use of pain medication.
- Presenting with vague symptoms and conditions.

Psychological/emotional

- Depression, anxiety or panic attacks.
- Evidence of self-harm.
- Evidence of attempted suicide.

Given that two women a week in the UK die as a result of domestic abuse, asking if a person is the victim of such abuse may be the most important question a midwife ever asks. However, the risk to the woman's safety and that of the midwife requires care when proceeding with the enquiry. In its resource manual for health professionals, the Department of Health (DH, 2000) recommends the following best practice.

- **See the woman on her own.** The presence of a partner or a relative may constrain discussion of domestic abuse and could place the woman in greater danger. The discussion should not take place in the presence of children.
- **Consider the need for an interpreter.** Some people may need someone else to be present (preferably of the same gender), either as an interpreter or as an advocate (particularly if the person has a learning disability), or for moral support. The person who is used as an interpreter should be independent and a professional. It is unacceptable to use family members or friends in this role, or to use staff who happen to have these skills but are not employed or trained to use them.
- **Ensure privacy.** The consultation should take place in a room in which confidentiality can be assured, and where the patient cannot be overheard or seen from outside the room, and where there will not be disturbance or interruption of the interview.
- **Emphasise confidentiality**, but be clear about its limits, and explain these to the woman. For example, if there are reasons to believe that a child may be at risk , the overriding duty will be to the child (*JD v East Berkshire Community Health NHS Trust* [2003]). Generally, it is considered good practice to respect a victim's confidentiality, and disclosure should only occur with consent. However, there may be circumstances where an immediate life or death situation, or an assessment of high risk of severe abuse, would justify disclosure to an appropriate source without consent. It is essentia,l therefore, that midwives are aware of information-sharing protocols for responding to domestic abuse with their employing Trusts.
- **Consider the welfare of any children.** Whenever there is a suspicion of domestic abuse, there should be awareness of the potential risks to any children. Children who have witnessed a violent episode may also need an immediate response to address their own needs and fears.

It can be seen that, for the safety of both the woman and the midwife, care needs to be taken when making a direct enquiry about domestic abuse.

Scenario

Diane is 35 and has recently undergone a caesarean section. Post-operatively, Diane has developed a fever and the wound is red and inflamed. She is also experiencing heavy blood losses.

Diane is visited by her partner on the third day. He insists she must come home. You explain to them both that it would not be in Diane's best interests to come home just yet as the wound is likely to be infected and that, should complications arise, she would be better off in hospital. There would be considerable difficulty in monitoring her in the community. In spite of this, Diane says she must obey her husband.

What actions could a midwife take in this situation?

Encouraging the woman to admit that she is a victim of domestic abuse is an important first step, but this can be a difficult step to take. It is therefore essential that, once the suspicion of abuse is confirmed, the midwife is able to offer appropriate advice and support.

Best practice recommends that, as a general rule, the duty of confidence to the woman should be maintained. The midwife will therefore be the only source of advice and information for the victim. It is essential that midwives are aware of the services available and the legal remedies that may be accessed by the victim to protect them from abuse.

Midwives must therefore have available information and contact details about local specialist agencies and refuge and national services, such as the National Domestic Violence Helpline, Women's Aid and Victim Support.

Scenario

Miss X is blind and lives with her brother, who has a learning disability. She is attending antenatal clinics. During one of the consultations, you notice a number of bruises on her shins and arms. You enquire as to the nature of the bruises. She tells you that her brother has been moving furniture around to make room for the baby and consequently she has to relearn how to navigate around her house.

Should you be concerned about her welfare? If so, in what way is she at significant risk?

Legal remedies for domestic abuse

The legal framework that seeks to protect and provide longer-term remedies for the victims of domestic abuse contains elements of both civil and criminal law. Midwives must have a general knowledge of the powers available under the law, in order to determine what support to give the victim and where the victim can obtain professional legal advice. As victims may also include children and vulnerable adults, knowledge of the law in these areas will enable better targeted referrals to specialist agencies.

Family Law Act 1996

The Family Law Act 1996 draws the civil remedies into one Act and makes them available to any family court. Part IV of the Act deals with domestic violence and details two types of order that can be used to protect those at risk of domestic abuse: *occupation orders*, which concern the right to occupy the family home; and *non-molestation orders*, which provide protection from violence or abuse.

To be eligible for the orders the victim must show that they are at risk from an associated person. An associated person could be a blood relative, a step-relative or someone who is or has been part of the same household. The term can also cover people who have been in an intimate relationship, whether or not they have lived together, people who have been 'parties to the same family proceedings' or individuals who have been legally connected by adoption. Therefore, an occupation order could be obtained by a sister against her brother or step-brother if they shared the same home.

The result of an occupation order is that the abuser is ousted from the home, allowing the victim of domestic abuse to remain there. The order can, however, have a variety of terms and conditions. These vary according to whether or not the person applying for the order is entitled to occupy the property and their relationship to the other party or parties.

A non-molestation order prevents the abuser from molesting the victim or a relevant child. It can prohibit particular actions and behaviour or molestation in general. In this respect, Parliament recognises that domestic abuse often transcends the use of physical force normally attributed to violence.

The court also has the power to make a non-molestation order without an application being made in other family proceedings. For example, if there are current proceedings for contact or residence orders (Children Act 1989, s8), the court will be able to make a non-molestation order for the benefit of a party to those proceedings, or a relevant child. A non-molestation order may last for a specified period or until a further order is made.

A child under 16 may apply for a non-molestation order with the leave of the court. Such leave will only be granted if the court is satisfied that the child is *Gillick* competent and therefore has sufficient understanding of the situation and the consequences of the order (*Gillick v West Norfolk and Wisbech AHA* [1986]).

For the abuser, the consequence of breaching an order, which is a criminal offence, is likely to be a custodial sentence.

CASE STUDY: *Consequence of breaching a non-molestation order*

In *G v C (Residence Order: Committal)* [1998], a young father, convicted of contempt of court following frequent breaches of a non-molestation order granted on the application of the mother of his children, was sentenced on appeal to eight months' imprisonment.

Protection from Harassment Act 1997

The major disadvantage of the powers available under the provisions of Part IV of the Family Law Act 1996 is that they rely on the victim taking action against the abuser. The Protection from Harassment Act 1997, however, allows the police to take criminal action against an abuser. This Act protects the victims of abuse by introducing two criminal offences of criminal harassment and putting people in fear of violence. These are supplemented by providing for civil restraining orders and damages to be awarded where they are broken. In terms of domestic abuse, the provisions are available to those victims of abuse who are not eligible for orders under the Family Law Act 1996.

Harassment is not defined in the Act but is based on the 'reasonable person' test – that is, a person ought to know that the course of conduct amounts to the harassment of another if a reasonable person in possession of the same information would think it was harassment. This objective test prevents a stalker from arguing that they were unaware of their obsession or did not think their behaviour was unusual. To be harassment, the course of conduct must have occurred on at least two occasions and can include speech.

In addition to a conviction, a restraining order may be imposed by the court, and this can include an exclusion or prohibited area into which the offender may not enter.

CASE STUDY: Restraining orders

In *R v Kasoar* [2002], a man was sentenced to 12 months' imprisonment for breach of a restraining order. The man had a relationship with a young woman that had broken down. Following the breakdown of the relationship, he parked his car outside the woman's place of work, was convicted of harassment and was made the subject of a restraining order. When she married another man, she was constantly followed from work to her home, with the result that her relationship with her husband was disrupted and ended in separation. The former boyfriend was arrested and convicted of breaching the restraining order.

Housing Act 1996

Victims of domestic abuse, who are generally women with children, are often concerned that they will be left homeless if they leave the family home to get away from their abuser. Although refuges are able to provide immediate assistance, the Housing Act 1996 allows those who are victims of domestic abuse to seek the help of their local housing authority. The authority is responsible for providing priority housing to homeless people as long as they are not intentionally homeless. A person fleeing from their home because of domestic abuse is considered homeless under the Housing Act 1996 and not intentionally homeless. This would be the case even if the person did not initially seek to make use of the legal remedies under the Family Law Act 1996.

CASE STUDY: Duty to rehouse victims of domestic abuse

In *Bond v Leicester City Council* [2001], a woman was considered intentionally homeless by the city council when she deliberately left her home after suffering violence and intimidation at the hands of her partner. The council argued that she should have protected herself by making use of the civil and criminal remedies available under the law before leaving home. The Court of Appeal held that this was wrong. The only test in determining homelessness was the likelihood of violence if they remained in the property. The woman was therefore not intentionally homeless and the council was responsible for rehousing her.

A further provision under section 145 of the Housing Act 1996 allows local housing authorities and social housing landlords to take action for repossession of a secure tenancy property where one partner has left because of domestic abuse and the court is satisfied that they are unlikely to return.

Causing or allowing death

The provisions under section 5 of the Domestic Violence, Crime and Victims Act 2004 created the offence of causing or allowing the death of a child or vulnerable adult. The offence is in response to a situation where a vulnerable person dies as a result of unlawful conduct, but it cannot be shown which of the accused caused the offence. Now, where such a person dies as a result of unlawful conduct and the death was caused by a member of the household, all members of the household (depending on age and capacity) will be liable if they caused or did not take reasonable steps to prevent the death. See Chapter 7 for more about cases involving violence against children.

Domestic homicide reviews

The Domestic Violence, Crime and Victims Act 2004 now requires that domestic homicide reviews are held by statutory bodies, including health authorities and PCTs, so that they can learn how such killings occurred and how they can be prevented in the future.

Safeguarding women from sexual abuse

Of all crimes, sexual crimes are viewed with particular revulsion because of their intimate nature and enduring effect on the victim. While such crimes are not unique to early twenty-first-century Britain, and numbers seem to be falling, offences often go unreported. Home Office statistics report that, in the year ending March 2005, the total number of recorded sexual offences in England and Wales was 60,900 – a 17 per cent increase on the previous year. However, numbers fell to 53,500 in the year ending March 2008, and again to 51,500 in the following year (Home Office, 2005; Home Office, 2009). Despite this fall in the numbers of reported incidents, it is argued that between 10 and 40 per cent of women are victims of unlawful sexual activity (Prescott, 2002). It is inevitable that midwives will provide care and support during pregnancy for women who have been sexually abused or are in an abusive relationship. It is essential, therefore, that you are aware of the key provisions of the Sexual Offences Act 2003 in order to recognise, and support, victims of unlawful sexual activity.

The development of sexual offences

Sexual offence laws have traditionally been derived from the Judaeo-Christian Church's condemnation of all sexual activity outside marriage. Historically, activities such as adultery and homosexuality were unlawful or considered deviant behaviour that needed treatment. Indeed, it was felt necessary to specifically exclude such behaviour from the legal definition of a mental disorder, and section 1(3) of the Mental Health Act 1983 stated that people must not be deemed to have a form of mental disorder *by reason only of promiscuity or other immoral conduct, sexual deviancy or dependence on alcohol or drugs.* In 2008, this overt exclusion was removed by the Mental Health Act 2007, with the government arguing that it was old-fashioned and no longer necessary, as in twenty-first-century Britain neither promiscuity nor other immoral conduct by itself was regarded as a mental disorder, nor was sexual orientation, so the exclusion was unnecessary.

Most sexual offences evolved during the nineteenth century and resulted in some of the crassest anomalies in the law from times when values and opinions used to prevail that have long since been abandoned. As seen by the changes to mental health law, reform has usually been achieved slowly, over time, in a piecemeal and unstructured fashion. For example, the Sexual Offences Act 1993 was enacted to abolish the legal presumption that a boy under the age of 14 was incapable of sexual intercourse. Prior to the passage of this Act, a boy would have been presumed to be physically incapable of penetrating a woman and therefore could not be considered guilty of rape.

CASE STUDY: Rape within marriage

The law of rape traditionally stated that sexual intercourse had to be unlawful and that was taken to mean outside marriage. In *R v R* [1992], the House of Lords overturned the principle in *Hale's History of the Pleas of the Crown 1736* (Emlyn, 1971), that a wife irrevocably consented to sexual intercourse with her husband on marriage. Their Lordships held that this assumption was no longer applicable in modern times when marriage was viewed as a partnership of equals. The Sexual Offences Act 1956 defined rape as *unlawful sexual intercourse with a woman who at the time of the intercourse does not consent to it*. The submission that 'unlawful' meant outside the bond of marriage was rejected and the word 'unlawful' was considered superfluous.

Sexual Offences Act 2003

The Sexual Offences Act 2003 had the broad aim of modernising the law regulating sexual activity. The focus of the modernisation was enhancing protection for children and vulnerable adults from unlawful sexual conduct (Home Office, 2002). This was achieved in three ways.

- It clarified and gave statutory meaning to key terms such as 'consent' and 'sexual'.
- It created specific offences that may be committed against children and the vulnerable.
- It enabled continuing protection from further sexual abuse by strengthening the notification requirements for sex offenders, managing high-risk offenders in the community through multi-agency public protection panels and creating a new civil prevention order.

Consent

Chapter 5 considered the role of consent in allowing a woman to express her autonomy by agreeing to the touching of her body for examination and treatment. Touching a woman without consent (or other operation of the law) is unlawful under the tort of trespass and crime of assault. Similarly, a valid consent is crucial to the lawfulness of sexual activity. The age of consent for all sexual activity is now 16 years (Sexual Offences Act 2003, s9), and there is no longer any difference between heterosexual and homosexual relationships.

There are two key elements to a valid consent.

- The person must be of sufficient age and understanding to be capable of making a choice.
- The person must make that choice freely and without constraint.

In a major change to the law relating to non-consensual sexual activity, it will no longer be possible for the defendant to argue that they genuinely believed that the victim had consented. The issue of consent is clarified further by sections 75 and 76 of the Sexual Offences Act 2003, which specify circumstances where the presumption must be that the victim did not consent. These include circumstances where:

- any person used or threatened violence against the complainant at the time of, or immediately before, the sexual activity began;
- any person caused the complainant to fear at the time of, or immediately before, the sexual act that violence was being used or would be used immediately against another person;
- the complainant was unlawfully detained at the time;
- the complainant was asleep or otherwise unconscious at the time;
- the complainant was unable to communicate consent to the defendant because of their physical disability, e.g. where a complainant is unable to communicate verbally or to nod or shake their head;
- any person administers or causes the complainant to take a substance, without the complainant's consent, which was capable of causing or enabling the complainant to be stupefied or overpowered at the time of the relevant act;
- the defendant intentionally deceived the complainant as to the nature or purpose of the relevant act;
- the defendant intentionally induced the complainant to consent to the relevant act by impersonating a person known personally to the complainant.

CASE STUDY: Sleeping woman

In *Melville v HM Advocate* [2006], a man appealed against his conviction for rape after being found guilty of having intercourse with a woman without her consent while she was asleep. Evidence from a witness suggested that, prior to the incident, Melville was behaving sexually towards the sleeping woman. The Court of Appeal upheld the rape conviction.

Clarifying consent in sexual activity by giving it a statutory definition that requires the defendant to have a reasonable belief that the victim consented, and specifying circumstances where a victim is presumed not to have consented, the Sexual Offences Act 2003 sends a clear signal to the public about situations where sexual activity is unlawful and encourages victims to bring cases to court. Where sexual activity takes place when consent is absent, a non-consensual sexual offence occurs regardless of the age of the victim.

Concept summary: Non-consensual sexual offences

Rape

This occurs where the defendant intentionally penetrates the vagina, anus or mouth of another person with his penis without consent and without reasonable belief of consent.

Assault by penetration

This occurs when the defendant intentionally penetrates the vagina or anus of another person with a part of their body (such as a finger) or anything else (such as a bottle), the penetration is sexual without consent and without reasonable belief of consent.

Concept summary continued

Sexual assault

This occurs when the defendant touches another person, the touching is sexual and without consent and without reasonable belief of consent.

Causing sexual activity without consent

This occurs when the defendant intentionally causes a person to engage in activity, the activity is sexual and without consent and without reasonable belief of consent. (For example, a victim is forced to carry out a sexual act involving their own person, such as self-masturbation, or engage in sexual activity with a third party, or engage in sexual activity with the offender such as when a woman forces a man to penetrate her.)

Female genital mutilation

It is estimated that 100 to 140 million girls and women worldwide are currently living with the consequences of female genital mutilation (FGM) (WHO, 2008).

In the UK, a report by FORWARD (2007) estimates that the prevalence of FGM in England and Wales is substantial and is on the increase. The practice is recognised internationally as a violation of human rights and constitutes an extreme form of discrimination against women (WHO, 2008). As it is nearly always carried out on minors, it is also a violation of the rights of children and breaches the significant harm threshold necessary for state intervention to protect children.

FGM includes procedures that intentionally alter or injure female genital organs for non-therapeutic purposes and that have no health benefits. The procedure is typically performed on girls aged between 4 and 13 years. However, in some cases FGM is performed on newborn infants or on young women prior to marriage or pregnancy.

There is a worldwide effort to eliminate such practices and midwives are in an ideal position to contribute to this global effort by taking appropriate action where they consider a girl or woman is at risk of being subject to the FGM procedure.

It is essential that midwives are aware of the law relating to FGM and make families aware that this practice is unlawful.

Female Genital Mutilation Act 2003

The Prohibition of Female Circumcision Act 1985 made FGM unlawful in England and Wales. However, there was evidence to suggest that people used a loophole in the 1985 Act to take young girls abroad temporarily to carry out FGM and, despite many girls being at risk in the UK, there have been few prosecutions. Only one general practitioner has been struck off the medical register for offering to perform FGM operations on females (*Ahmed v General Medical Council* [2001]).

The Female Genital Mutilation Act 2003 came into force in March 2004. It repealed the 1985 Act (now reflecting WHO's preferred terminology of genital mutilation rather than circumcision), and offers greater protection to those at risk of FGM. The term 'girl' refers to females of all ages. Under the provisions of this Act, it is an offence for any person to:

- excise, infibulate or otherwise mutilate the whole or any part of a girl's labia majora, labia minora or clitoris;

- aid, abet, counsel or procure the performance by another person of any of those acts on that other person's body;
- aid, abet, counsel or procure a person to excise, infibulate or otherwise mutilate the whole or any part of her own labia majora, labia minora or clitoris. (This means that, while it is not an offence for a girl to mutilate her own genitalia, it is an offence to assist a girl to mutilate her own genitalia (Female Genital Mutilation Act 2003, s2).)

The 2003 Act also introduced the concept of *extraterritoriality*, making it a criminal offence to take any girl who is a UK national or UK permanent resident to any other country for FGM. In addition, the new law increased the penalty for carrying out FGM, or arranging to have FGM carried out, to 14 years' imprisonment or a fine or both.

Exceptions under the Female Genital Mutilation Act 2003

There are often few practical distinctions between procedures involved in carrying out FGM and those involved in carrying out legitimate surgery. Therefore, under section 2(a) of the 2003 Act, no offence is committed by a registered medical practitioner who performs a surgical operation on a girl that is necessary for her physical or mental health. However, when assessing a girl's mental health, no account can be taken of any belief that the operation is needed as a matter of custom or ritual. Therefore, an FGM operation could not legally occur on the grounds that a girl's mental health would suffer if she did not conform to the custom of her community.

A further exception under section 2(b) of the Act allows a surgical operation on a girl who is in any stage of labour, or has just given birth, for purposes connected with the labour or birth. This operation may be carried out by an approved person who can be a registered medical practitioner, a registered midwife or a person undergoing a course of training with a view to becoming such a practitioner or midwife. However, midwives must note that it is unlawful to reinfibulate a woman following the birth of her baby.

Female genital mutilation and child protection

Female genital mutilation can cause significant harm and suffering to the girl involved. It is important that midwives work closely with other agencies to safeguard the health and well-being of girls who they reasonably believe are likely to be, or have been, subjected to FGM.

Where a girl has already undergone FGM and this comes to the midwife's attention, a referral should be made to social services or the police Child Abuse Investigation Team. The circumstances of the case, such as how, where and when the procedure was performed and its implications for other female children in the family, will be investigated. If the circumstances fall within the provisions of the Female Genital Mutilation Act 2003, the police will investigate and a prosecution will be considered.

In any cases of FGM relating to minors it is important to consider the welfare of the child. Although the Children Act 1989 does not specifically mention FGM, it is covered as it meets the significant harm criteria. FGM differs from other forms of child abuse as it is considered part of the culture and religion of many people and is not perceived as being wrong or an act of abuse. Parents are often under pressure from older relatives to agree to FGM. It therefore might not be appropriate to remove a girl from an otherwise caring family. However, it is the welfare of the child that is always paramount and any decision must take this welfare principle into account.

If a local authority has reason to believe that a child is likely to suffer significant harm as a result of FGM, it must consider an investigation under section 47 of the

Children Act 1989. A local authority must treat as serious all allegations of abuse reported to them by midwives (*Re E (Children) (Care Proceedings: Social Work Practice)* [2000]).

It is essential that midwives are aware of the law relating to FGM in order to provide advice and assistance to those in their care who may be affected by this unlawful practice.

Protecting vulnerable women from unsuitable midwives and carers

Vulnerable women can be subjected to abuse in a variety of settings, and it is particularly shocking when the perpetrator is someone who has a duty of care.

Abuse of a position of trust

Where an adult in a position of trust, such as a midwife or a teacher, has a sexual relationship with a child under 18, the law sets aside the child's consent to the sexual activity and the adult is deemed to have committed an offence under the Sexual Offences Act 2003. As well as offences designed to protect minors from sexual exploitation, the Act also creates a similar series of offences that may be categorised as breaches of a relationship of care (see the concept summary below). The provisions are designed to protect those with a learning disability or mental disorder who have capacity to consent but who are vulnerable to exploitation, and who may agree to sexual activity because they are familiar with, or dependent on, their carers. These offences criminalise matters that have traditionally been dealt with by regulatory bodies such as the NMC.

Concept summary: Offences against persons with a mental disorder

Under the heading 'Care workers for persons with a mental disorder', sections 38–41 of the Sexual Offences Act 2003 list the following offences:

- sexual activity with a person with a mental disorder;
- causing or inciting sexual activity with a person with a mental disorder;
- sexual activity in the presence of a person with a mental disorder;
- causing a person with a mental disorder to watch a sexual act.

The 2003 Act defines a care worker very broadly and includes health and social care workers who provide support in care homes, hospitals, the person's own home and day centres. This also includes a wide range of people who support people with a learning disability or mental disorder, such as support workers, therapists, receptionists and complementary therapists.

CASE STUDY: Health worker put on sex offenders register

A health worker employed at a psychiatric hospital in North Wales admitted four charges of engaging in sexual activity with a person with a mental disorder when he had an affair with a woman who was a patient at the hospital where he worked. He was jailed for two years at Mold Crown Court and put on the sex offenders' register for 10 years (Bellis, 2005).

The Vetting and Barring Scheme

Following the murders of Jessica Chapman and Holly Wells in 2002 and the subsequent Bichard Inquiry (2004), the Safeguarding Vulnerable Groups Act 2006 was passed to ensure a more robust system to safeguard those at risk. Bichard recommended that new arrangements be introduced requiring those who wish to work with children or vulnerable adults in England, Wales or Northern Ireland to be registered. The Vetting and Barring Scheme (VBS) confirms that there is no known reason why an individual should not work with these clients.

Scotland has its own VBS under the Protection of Vulnerable Groups (Scotland) Act 2007 and a Central Barring Unit, which considers individuals for listing on the children's and adults' lists and maintains those lists. Both schemes share information and recognise each other's barring lists. Generally, an individual barred anywhere within the UK will also be barred across the rest of the UK. When an individual's name is placed on the barred list, that person is not able to work with vulnerable adults and/or children until his or her name is removed from the list.

The Independent Safeguarding Authority (ISA) now assesses the suitability of those who want to work with vulnerable people in partnership with the Criminal Records Bureau (CRB). The ISA maintains a children barred list and an adult barred list for people barred from engaging in what are now called regulated activities.

In June 2010, the new coalition government, in response to growing pressure from parents, authors and civil liberties groups who were concerned about the scope of the VBS, decided to delay its implementation pending a review, which will seek to scale back the scheme to common-sense proportions.

Regulated activities

Regulated activities cover a wide range of activities that provide the opportunity for close contact with vulnerable adults. They include any activity involving frequent, intensive or overnight contact. Some activities are regulated because of their nature and this includes providing care and treatment. So activities that allow frequent or intensive contact with vulnerable adults in a hospital, care home or clinic are regulated activities. This definition clearly includes midwives and student midwives, who will be required to register with the ISA and subject themselves to the vetting process.

Controlled activities

Controlled activities give some opportunity for contact with children or vulnerable adults, but are more remote than regulated activities. Controlled activities cover frequent or intensive support work in health settings, further education settings and adult social care settings, such as the work of cleaners, caretakers, receptionists, catering staff and so on. IThey also include those working for a specific organisation, such as an NHS Trust, with frequent access to sensitive records about children and vulnerable adults.

Inclusion on the barred list

There are a number of routes to inclusion on the barred lists.

- Automatic inclusion with no right of representation or appeal covers the most serious offences listed by the 2006 Act, including serious sexual offences against children and vulnerable adults. A person is automatically placed on the barred list and there is no right to make representation or to appeal because there can be no mitigating circumstances that might explain why these offences have been committed.

- Automatic inclusion with a right to representation and appeal covers certain offences, such as theft or fraud, which might indicate that there is a probable risk of harm to children or vulnerable adults but not necessarily in every conceivable case. A person is immediately placed on the barred list following a conviction or caution, but is entitled to make representation as to why their name should be removed from the list.
- Inclusion based on relevant conduct means that a person will be included on the barred list on the basis that they engaged in behaviour that might have harmed a vulnerable adult. This includes having sexual material relating to children, having sexually explicit images depicting violence against human beings, and conduct of a sexual nature involving a vulnerable adult. The person has the opportunity to make relevant representation before they are included on the list.
- Inclusion at the discretion of the ISA may occur where information such as unproven allegations from former employers, professional bodies or members of the public give cause for concern. Before a barring decision is made, the individual is given the information on which the decision is based and the opportunity to explain their case.

C H A P T E R   S U M M A R Y

- Identifying a vulnerable adult and a victim of abuse is a key duty for a midwife.
- In 2002, the Department of Health defined a vulnerable adult as:

  a person aged 18 years or over, who is in receipt of or may be in need of community care services by reason of mental or other disability, age or illness and who is or may be unable to take care of him or herself, or unable to protect him or herself against significant harm or exploitation.

  This definition was followed by a commitment to protect such individuals.
- There are different categories of abuse, including physical, sexual, psychological, financial or material abuse, and neglect.
- Forced marriage is a form of abuse, and is against the law. Midwives may well come across young women who have been married against their will.
- In the UK, two women a week die as a result of domestic abuse. Midwives should be aware of signs that might indicate that a woman is being abused, and should give the woman the privacy and the opportunity to answer questions about possible abuse.
- The Sexual Offences Act 2003 has modernised the law relating to sexual behaviour and has clarified the issue of consent in sexual relationships.
- Midwives should make sure they know who to inform if they suspect a woman in their care is the victim of abuse.
- Female genital mutilation is a form of abuse that is still culturally sanctioned in some parts of the world, although it is illegal in the UK. Some female infants as well as young girls may be at risk of this mutilation. Midwives may also find themselves caring for pregnant women who have been mutilated.
- Occasionally, health professionals, including midwives, can be abusers. This means that stringent safeguards are in position to protect the public. All midwives must now be assessed by the Independent Safeguarding Authority (ISA) to ensure that they will not abuse the trust of the women in their care.

Knowledge review

Having completed the chapter, how would you now rate your knowledge of the following topics?

	Good	Adequate	Poor
1. The definition of abuse and the concept of 'significant harm'.			
2. The role of the law in protecting vulnerable adults and victims of domestic abuse.			
3. The main provisions of the Sexual Offences Act 2003 as they relate to pregnant and vulnerable women.			
4. The policies that protect women from unsuitable midwives and carers.			

Where you're not confident in your knowledge of a topic, what will you do next?

Further reading

For a more in-depth consideration of the topics covered in this chapter, we recommend the following texts:

Department of Health (DH) (2002) No Secrets. London: DH. Available online at **www.doh. gov.uk/en/PublicationsandstatisticsPublicationsPolicyAndGuidance/DH_4008486**.

Stobart, E (2007) *Dealing with Cases of Forced Marriage: Practice guidance for health professionals*. London: Foreign and Commonwealth Office and Department of Health. Available online at **www.dh.gov.uk/en/Publications/PublicationsPolicyAnd Guidance/DH_084449**.

Law Commission (1992) *Report on Domestic Violence and Occupation of the Family Home*, Report No. 207: London: The Stationery Office.

For an in-depth review of sexual offences law that includes the historical development of the laws we recommend:

Laws, E and **Lees, P** (2007) *The Sexual Offences Referencer: A practitioner's guide to indictments and sentencing*. Oxford: Oxford University Press.

Useful websites

www.cps.gov.uk/news/fact_sheets/sexual_offences Crown Prosecution Service site that has the CPS's web factsheet on sexual offences.

www.dh.gov.uk/en/PublicationsandstatisticsPublicationsPolicyAndGuidance/DH_4126161 Department of Health site that has resources on domestic abuse and the resource manual for health professionals.

www.homeoffice.gov.uk/rds/pdfs04/dpr30.pdf Home Office site that carries Home Office information-sharing guidance for practitioners.

Chapter 12

Law, reproduction and the status of the unborn child

Chapter aims

After reading this chapter, you will be able to:

- outline the law relating to the termination of pregnancy;
- explain the rights bestowed on an unborn child;
- describe how surrogacy is regulated in the UK;
- discuss the regulation of assisted conception by the Human Fertilisation and Embryology Act 1990 (as amended).

Introduction

This chapter considers the regulation of treatments to terminate pregnancy and assist couples to conceive. It outlines the law on abortion and discusses the legal status of the unborn child. Following on from this, it looks at the role of the law in regulating assisted conception and addresses the practical dilemmas that arise from these treatments.

In 2008, there were 708,711 live births in England and Wales, but some 195,296 pregnancies were terminated (DH/ONS, 2009). Abortion gives rise to a number of moral and legal dilemmas, which are also regulated by the law.

The Human Fertilisation and Embryology Authority (HFEA) suggests that infertility is the most common reason for women aged 20–45 to see their GP, after pregnancy itself. It is estimated that infertility affects about one in six couples in the UK; although many of these will become pregnant naturally, a significant number will require medical assistance to conceive. Assisted conception techniques such as in vitro fertilisation and surrogacy give rise to a number of legal dilemmas that are now regulated by law.

Abortion

There is no legal definition of the term 'abortion'. Douglas (1993) suggests that it is any treatment to terminate pregnancy.

Activity 12.1	Group work

In a group make a list of reasons why you think it is necessary to regulate the treatment that terminates pregnancy.

Please do not move on to the next part until you are ready for the answer.

Your list is likely to have included reasons based on the right to life of the unborn child and the general principle of the sanctity of all life, and may also have included fundamental moral and religious arguments against abortion.

Abortion remains a controversial subject more than 40 years after the Abortion Act 1967 liberalised the law relating to the termination of pregnancy. The horns of the dilemma, as indicated by your list, continue to be the right of a woman to seek an abortion against the right of the child to be born alive. Both pro-choice and pro-life groups are dissatisfied with the current law. There are calls for change, with pro-life lobby groups asking for a reduction in the time limit on abortion and a statutory cooling-off period before a woman has an abortion. Pro-choice lobbyists are demanding less regulation and increased choice for women by allowing health professionals other than doctors to terminate pregnancies. The debate shows little sign of abating: amendments to the Abortion Act 1967 were put to Parliament on no fewer than four different occasions in 2009 alone.

The law's early focus on terminating a pregnancy was based on the sanctity of life. Procuring a miscarriage has been a crime in England and Wales since 1803 under Ellenborough's Act. Prior to that, abortion was lawful provided it was carried out before the woman felt the foetus move ('quickening'), when it was believed that the soul entered the body. In 1803, the law changed and abortion became a criminal offence from the time of conception. Under the 1803 Act, an abortion performed after quickening carried the death penalty. The relatively lesser penalties of fine, imprisonment, whipping or transportation were prescribed for abortion before quickening. Now, under the provisions of the Offences Against the Person Act 1861, section 58, it is a criminal offence to administer drugs or use instruments to procure an abortion:

> Every woman, being with child, who, with intent to procure her own miscarriage, shall unlawfully administer to herself any poison or other noxious thing, or shall unlawfully use any instrument or other means whatsoever . . . and whosoever, with intent to procure the miscarriage of any woman, whether she be or be not with child, shall unlawfully administer to her or cause to be taken by her any poison or other noxious thing, or shall unlawfully use any instrument or other means whatsoever . . . shall be guilty of felony.

It is, therefore, an offence for a pregnant woman to procure her own miscarriage and a person who unlawfully procures the miscarriage of any woman will be guilty of the offence whether or not the woman is pregnant. If the woman dies as a result of an unlawful termination of pregnancy, the charge becomes one of manslaughter.

CASE STUDY: A criminal abortion

In *R v Buck* (1964), two people were charged, one with manslaughter and the other with being an accessory to manslaughter, after a criminal abortion that resulted in the death of a woman whom the second defendant had counselled and procured.

The court held both were guilty because, where death results from a criminal abortion, there must be at least a conviction for manslaughter, as there is always a risk of death in a criminal abortion, and a person who procures another to commit a criminal abortion that results in death must also be guilty of being an accessory to manslaughter.

CASE STUDY: A surgeon charged with abortion

In *R v Dixon* [1995], a consultant surgeon was charged with unlawfully procuring a miscarriage under the Offences Against the Person Act 1861 when he decided to continue with a hysterectomy even after discovering an 11-week foetus in the womb (Dyer, 2002).

The surgeon was found not guilty of the offence, but was later reprimanded by his regulatory body, the General Medical Council, after acknowledging that he had made the wrong decision but saying that he had been acting in what he thought was the patient's best interests.

Infant Life (Preservation) Act 1929

The Infant Life (Preservation) Act 1929 closed a loophole in the law where a child was killed in the course of being born, and made it an offence to kill a child capable of being born alive before it had an existence independent of its mother. The Act created a presumption that a foetus of 28 weeks' gestation is capable of being born alive. This does not, however, lower the limit on a child capable of being born alive and the courts have considered the application of the Act to less mature foetuses. In *Rance v Mid Downs HA* [1991], the court held that a 26-week-old foetus was a child capable of being born alive, because after birth it existed as a living breathing child. In *C v S (Foetus: Unmarried Father)* [1988], the court held that a foetus of 18 to 21 weeks was not a child capable of being born alive.

CASE STUDY: Child destruction

A woman was convicted on the rare charge of child destruction after visiting a back-street abortionist to terminate her seven and a half month-old foetus (Britten, 2007). She was given a 12-month suspended sentence and is believed to be the first expectant mother to be convicted under the Infant Life (Preservation) Act 1929, even though she has never admitted what she did and no body was ever found.

CASE STUDY continued

The woman was thought to have fallen pregnant in July 2005 while having an affair with a taxi driver. Prosecutors believe she travelled to Liverpool in February 2006 for an abortion because the baby was illegitimate. She later claimed she had miscarried, but gave several different versions of events, none of which was able to be confirmed.

She denied child destruction, but the jury took only 47 minutes to convict her.

Lawful termination of pregnancy

To be lawful a termination of pregnancy must be covered by the provisions of the Abortion Act 1967, which creates a defence to the established criminal offences of unlawfully procuring a miscarriage under section 58 of the Offences Against the Person Act 1861, or child destruction under section 1(1) of the Infant Life (Preservation) Act 1929.

The Abortion Act 1967 operates by providing a defence to these charges when the conditions set out in its provisions are met. It replaces a common law defence established by *R v Bourne* [1939], where an eminent surgeon performed an abortion on a 14-year-old girl who had been made pregnant as a result of a violent rape by a gang of soldiers, and who had attempted suicide as a result. The judge ruled that Bourne had acted in the belief that the abortion would preserve the life of the mother. In his summing up, the judge focused on the word 'unlawful' in section 58 of the Offences Against the Person Act 1861, arguing that the word was to highlight that there must be lawful reasons for procuring a miscarriage. The jury decided that one of these reasons was to preserve the life of the woman and acquitted Bourne. Subsequent decisions by the courts resulted in a broader interpretation, allowing abortions to preserve the mental and physical health as well as the life of the mother.

The common law defence continues to operate as the Abortion Act 1967, which does not extend to Northern Ireland.

The Abortion Act 1967

Since the introduction of the Abortion Act 1967, more than 20 attempts at reform have been proposed, but none succeeded until the passage of the Human Fertilisation and Embryology Act 1990 allowed for a full debate on the issue of abortion law (Douglas, 1993). Section 37 of the 1990 Act introduced four principal amendments to the Abortion Act 1967:

- enlarging the grounds for abortion contained in section 1(1) of the Abortion Act 1967;
- providing a defence to the Infant Life (Preservation) Act 1929, removing the time limit it imposed;
- setting an upper time limit of 24 weeks for the first ground for abortion concerning risk of injury to the physical or mental health of the pregnant woman or any existing children of her family, but removing any time limit for the other grounds (Abortion Act 1967, s1(1));
- clarifying the law on selective reduction in assisted conception.

The amended Abortion Act 1967 states that a person shall not be guilty of an offence under the law relating to abortion when a pregnancy is terminated by a registered medical practitioner, if two registered medical practitioners are of the opinion, formed in good faith, that:

- the pregnancy has not exceeded its twenty-fourth week and that the continuance of the pregnancy would involve risk, greater than if the pregnancy were terminated, of injury to the physical or mental health of the pregnant woman or any existing children of her family; or
- the termination is necessary to prevent grave permanent injury to the physical or mental health of the pregnant woman; or
- the continuance of the pregnancy would involve risk to the life of the pregnant woman, greater than if the pregnancy were terminated; or
- there is a substantial risk that if the child were born it would suffer from such physical or mental abnormalities as to be seriously handicapped.

The amendments introduced by the Human Fertilisation and Embryology Act 1990 do not confer on women a right to abortion. Doctors are the gatekeepers of the Abortion Act 1967 and they may grant or refuse an abortion. In *R v Smith* [1974], the Court of Appeal held that the Abortion Act 1967 places a great social responsibility on the shoulders of the medical profession as, before the procedure, two doctors must agree in good faith that one or more of the criteria set out in the 1967 Act apply. There is no requirement that any doctor in particular signs the certificate of opinion, or that they must see and examine the woman. In extreme cases the court may call into question the good faith of the doctor.

CASE STUDY: Not in good faith

In *R v Smith* [1974], a doctor carried out only a limited examination of the woman, took no medical history and made no further enquiries or investigations, yet agreed to do the abortion for cash. The jury concluded that the doctor had not formed his opinion in good faith and convicted him for procuring a miscarriage.

The 1967 Act also requires that the termination of a pregnancy be performed by a registered medical practitioner (Abortion Act 1967, s1(1)). The issue of the involvement of other health professionals in the termination of pregnancy was considered by the House of Lords in *Royal College of Nursing v DHSS* [1981], where they held that the requirement should be broadly accepted to take account of the health team. As long as the procedure is considered acceptable medical practice under the supervision of the doctor, the Abortion Act 1967 applied, and midwives and nurses as well as doctors were afforded a defence.

Post-coital contraception

Women now have a further option for family planning with the introduction of post-coital contraception, using drugs (morning-after pill) or an intrauterine device (IUD). Questions were initially raised over whether such measures amounted to a procurement of a miscarriage within the meaning of the Offences Against the Person Act 1861. If this were the case, administering the morning-after pill would have to comply with the provisions of the Abortion Act 1967.

The issue was clarified by the courts, which held that these techniques prevented an embryo implanting in the womb and without implantation there could be no miscarriage (*R (on the application of Smeaton) v Secretary of State for Health* [2002]).

> **CASE STUDY: No miscarriage without implantation**
>
> In *R v Dhingra* (1991), the court dismissed a charge under section 58 of the Offences Against the Person Act 1861 against a doctor who fitted an IUD to a woman 11 days after intercourse had taken place.
>
> In *R (on the application of Smeaton) v Secretary of State for Health* [2002], the sale of the morning-after pill without a prescription was also deemed not to be in contravention of the Offences Against the Person Act 1861, section 58, as the court found that the term 'miscarriage' was an ordinary word of the English language, to be defined in the light of current scientific and medical knowledge as a termination of pregnancy after implantation. As the morning-after pill prevents implantation there was no miscarriage.

Time limits and grounds for abortion

Section 1(1) of the Abortion Act 1967 provides four grounds for legal abortion:

- risk to the physical or mental health of the mother or existing children;
- prevention of grave permanent physical or mental injury;
- risk to the life of the mother;
- a substantial risk that the child would suffer from physical or mental abnormalities so as to be seriously handicapped.

Risk to the physical or mental health of the mother or existing children

These grounds are the most common for seeking an abortion. In 2008, some 98 per cent of the 195,296 abortions that took place in England and Wales were authorised for this reason (DH/ONS, 2009). These are also the only grounds to have a time limit imposed, which is currently 24 weeks. This represents Parliament's view of the stage of development where a foetus was capable of surviving if born, and was introduced in 1991 by the Human Fertilisation and Embryology Act 1990 (Kennedy and Grubb, 1998).

Within the last few years, pro-life groups have argued that developments in medical technology mean that a foetus becomes viable at a much lower stage of development and there have been several calls for the time limit to be reduced. In 2006, the Termination of Pregnancy Ten Minute Rule Bill sought to reduce the limit from 24 to 21 weeks and introduce a 10-day cooling off period from the time of the request for an abortion to the time the procedure was carried out, in order to enable counselling. The Ten Minute Rule Bill, which is more a device to raise issues and generate debate and rarely becomes law, was defeated in the House of Commons.

The three remaining grounds for abortion have no time limit. Until 1991 the time limit for all terminations of pregnancy was imposed by the provisions of the Infant Life (Preservation) Act 1929, which made it unlawful to terminate a foetus capable of being born alive. However, the amendment introduced by the Human Fertilisation and Embryology Act 1990 separated the Abortion Act 1967 from the Infant Life (Preservation) Act 1929. The 1967 Act now provides that no offence under the 1929 Act shall be committed by a registered medical practitioner who terminates a pregnancy in accordance with the provisions of this Act (at section 5(1)). This effectively removes the 28-week time limit for abortion from the remaining three grounds and, in law, a termination of pregnancy could occur right to term. Although in practice this is rarely the case, in 2006 some 136 terminations occurred beyond 24 weeks (DH/ONS, 2009). It was Parliament's view that a time limit on abortions should not be imposed where serious dangers to the health of the mother existed (*Hansard*, 1990).

Substantial risk of serious handicap

A pregnancy may be terminated where two doctors certify that there is a substantial risk that the child will suffer from such physical or mental abnormalities so as to be seriously handicapped. There has been no time limit on these grounds for abortion since 1991, so a termination of pregnancy could occur for foetal abnormality right up to term. Again, in practice this is rarely the case and the main source of controversy concerning these grounds relates to the interpretation of the terms 'substantial risk' and 'seriously handicapped'.

'Substantial risk' is a difficult term to quantify and the 1967 Act and its regulations offer little guidance. Of equal concern is that what amounts to a serious handicap is difficult to interpret and must be a question of law for the courts. In 2008, chromosomal abnormalities were reported for about a third of cases on these grounds, with congenital malformations in about half of cases. The most common of these were of the nervous system and the musculoskeletal system. Down's syndrome was the most commonly reported chromosomal abnormality and accounted for a fifth of all cases.

Kennedy and Grubb (1998) argue that, provided the condition is not trivial or easily correctible, such as a harelip, or merely leads the child to being disadvantaged, the law will allow doctors scope for determining the seriousness of a condition. They further argue that, to be a serious handicap, the child would have to have a physical or mental disability that would cause significant suffering or long-term impairment of their ability to function in society.

CASE STUDY: Cleft palate as grounds for termination

In *Jepson v The Chief Constable of West Mercia Police Constabulary* [2003], a doctor performed a late abortion on the grounds that the child had a serious handicap, namely a cleft lip and palate. Jepson argued that such a condition did not amount to a serious handicap and only required routine corrective surgery. However, the police and the CPS decided not to prosecute on the grounds that they were satisfied that the doctors involved in the termination had acted in good faith. The decision reflects the degree of discretion the law affords doctors in relation to the termination of pregnancy, and has led some to question whether the decision to grant access to an abortion should still be in the hands of doctors (Grear, 2004).

Wrongful life

The existence of liberal abortion laws has led to a challenge in court arguing that doctors and midwives owe a duty to a baby to offer the mother an abortion if they have evidence that the baby is likely to be born with a handicap. If such a duty existed, a baby born with deformities would be entitled to recover damages for negligence.

However, in *McKay v Essex HA* [1982], a baby born disabled as a result of an infection of rubella, suffered by her mother while the child was in her womb, failed in her bid for damages for wrongful life. The child and mother alleged that, but for the negligence of the doctor and midwives, the mother would have had an abortion to terminate the life of the child. The court found that there was no legal obligation under the Abortion Act 1967 to the foetus to terminate its life, and the child's claim was contrary to public policy as a violation of the sanctity of human life, as it would mean regarding the life of a handicapped child as not only less valuable than the life of a normal child, but so much less valuable that it was not worth preserving.

Rights of the father

Only a woman has the right to seek an abortion. She takes the risks, so her interests should outweigh those of the father (*C v S (Foetus: Unmarried Father)* [1988]). There is no requirement to notify the father and the father has no right of veto.

> **CASE STUDY: Father objects to abortion**
>
> In *Paton v British Pregnancy Advisory Service Trustees* [1979], a woman sought an abortion and two doctors certified, in accordance with section 1 of the Abortion Act 1967, that the continuance of her pregnancy would involve risk of injury to her physical or mental health. Her husband, who had not been consulted, objected and sought an injunction restraining her from having the abortion.
>
> The court dismissed his application and found that a husband has no enforceable legal or equitable right to prevent his wife from having a legal abortion.

Legal status of the unborn child

Under English law, an unborn child has no legal rights until it is born alive (*Paton v British Pregnancy Advisory Service Trustees* [1979]). An unborn child cannot sue or recover damages and, in *R v Tait* [1990], a threat to a pregnant woman to kill her unborn child was held not to be a threat to kill a third person under the Offences Against the Person Act 1861, section 16, because a foetus is not a person distinct from its mother. However, once born alive, a child can retrospectively apply its rights back into the womb.

> **CASE STUDY: Retrospective rights of the unborn child**
>
> In *Re Attorney General's Reference (No. 3 of 1994)* [1998], a man stabbed a pregnant woman who subsequently gave birth prematurely. The child, who had been injured by the stabbing in the womb, died some days later. The House of Lords held that, although the foetus was not a living person at the time, it was reasonable to charge the man with manslaughter once the child had been born alive.

At civil law the Congenital Disability (Civil Liability) Act 1976 allows children born suffering disabilities caused by medical negligence before birth to sue for a breach of duty of care, even though they were not persons in the eyes of the law when the injury took place.

> **CASE STUDY: Negligence before birth**
>
> In *B v Islington HA* [1993], a baby was born with disabilities caused by negligent treatment of the mother during pregnancy.
>
> The court found that a child born suffering disabilities caused by medical negligence before birth can sue for breach of duty of care since, although not a

person in the eyes of the law when the injury took place, an unborn child is clothed with all the rights of action when born alive that it would have had if in existence at the date of the accident to its mother.

Conflict between a mother and an unborn child

As an unborn child has no legal personality, any conflict of interests between the mother and the foetus is resolved in favour of the mother. The Infant Life (Preservation) Act 1929, section 1, makes it an offence to destroy the life of a child capable of being born alive, unless the act was necessary to preserve the life of the pregnant woman.

In terms of medical treatment, the law in principle is clear. As a capable adult, a pregnant woman has an absolute right to refuse medical treatment irrespective of the risks to her own life or that of her unborn child (see also the case study about refusal of a caesarean section on page 76 of Chapter 5).

Reforming the legal status of the unborn child

The only way to resolve this dilemma in favour of the unborn child would be to change the legal status of the foetus. The courts have made it clear that such a change is beyond their authority and would have to come from Parliament (*Re F (In Utero)* [1988]).

In some American states it is an offence to refuse a caesarean and a woman from Utah was charged with murder when her child died as a result of her refusal of treatment (Watson, 2004). It is very unlikely that such a law would be introduced in the UK. The key question for Parliament to address would be whether the status of an unborn child should change when a woman goes into labour.

Notification and registration requirements

There is a legal duty on the midwife attending a woman in labour to notify the PCT for the area of the birth and whether the baby was born alive or dead. The requirement applies to babies born after the twenty-fourth week of pregnancy in hospital or in the community. The notification must be posted within 36 hours on a pre-paid card to the PCT (NHS Act 2006, s269).

Registration of births

It is the duty of the baby's father or mother to give the Registrar, within 42 days of the birth (21 days in Scotland), information about the birth to allow it to be registered. If the father or mother does not do this, it will fall to any other person present at the birth to do so and this can include the midwife (Births and Deaths Registration Act 1953, s2).

Notification of deaths

For the purpose of the Births and Deaths Registration Act 1953, a baby born at any stage of pregnancy who breathes or shows other signs of life after complete expulsion from its mother is born alive; if the baby dies after birth, the birth and the death must both be registered.

A stillborn child is defined by law as a child born after the twenty-fourth week of pregnancy that did not at any time after being completely delivered from its mother breathe or show any other signs of life (Still-Birth (Definition) Act 1992, s1). The procedure for the registration of a stillborn child is set out in the Births and Deaths Registration Act 1953, section 11. It requires that, in the event of a stillbirth, one of the following must sign a certificate stating that the child was not born alive:

- a registered medical practitioner who was present at the birth or has examined the body of the child;
- a practising midwife who was so present or has examined the body.

A stillborn baby cannot be buried or cremated until a certificate has been obtained from the Registrar or an order for burial has been obtained from the Coroner. A midwife's signature on a stillbirth certificate is sufficient to allow the Registrar or Coroner to order the burial of a stillborn child. However, under the Cremation Act 1902 and its regulations, although a registered midwife may sign a stillbirth certificate, only a certificate signed by a registered medical practitioner will suffice in obtaining the crematorium's medical referee's permission to cremate a stillborn child.

Where a baby born before the twenty-fourth week of pregnancy does not breathe or show signs of life after complete expulsion from its mother, in law this is neither a live birth nor a stillbirth and need not be registered. There is also no legal duty under burial law to bury or cremate babies born dead before 24 weeks' gestation, currently the legal age of viability. There is, however, nothing to prevent NHS Trusts making arrangements for the burial or cremation of babies born dead before the legal age of viability.

Concealing the birth of a child

It is an offence for a mother or any person present at the birth, including the midwife, to conceal the birth of a child, whether it is born alive or stillborn, as illustrated by this case study.

CASE STUDY: Babies in the attic

A woman admitted three charges of concealing the births of her babies when they were discovered in bags in the attic of her previous home 30 years later. She admitted keeping the pregnancies hidden from her family and delivered the babies herself when her children were at school. She said that each baby was stillborn and she hid their bodies out of a misguided sense of shame and fear of rejection. She received a 12-month community rehabilitation order from the court (Savill, 2005).

Assisted conception: surrogacy

The Warnock Committee defines surrogacy as a practice whereby one woman carries a child for another with the intention that the child should be handed over at birth (DHSS, 1984, p42).

Two types of surrogacy arrangement have been identified. There is partial surrogate motherhood, where the surrogate's ovum is impregnated with the commissioning father's sperm, usually through intercourse or artificial insemination. This type of surrogacy is now more commonly referred to as straight surrogacy or traditional surrogacy.

The second type is called full surrogacy, womb leasing or gestational surrogacy, as it involves the implantation of the commissioning couple's embryo into the surrogate through IVF.

Activity 12.2 — *Reflection and group work*

- In a group consider whether any or all forms of surrogacy arrangement should be permitted in the UK.
- List what you consider to be the benefits and risks of surrogacy.

As this activity is based on your own views and reflections, no outline answer is given at the end of the chapter.

Acceptability of surrogacy

At the time of the Warnock Committee report (DHSS, 1984), the public's view was firmly against surrogacy, particularly surrogacy for convenience and paid surrogacy. Now, in twenty-first century Britain, the attitude towards the practice has softened. After initially recommending that doctors have no involvement with surrogacy arrangements, the British Medical Association now sees it as a valuable reproductive option of last resort (Craft, 1996).

The Human Fertilisation and Embryology Act 2008 also allows the commissioning couple to become registered as the parents of a child born as a result of a surrogacy arrangement, if they meet the requirements of the parental order. From April 2010, this has included same-sex couples, whether or not in a civil partnership, as well as married and unmarried couples.

Despite public, medical and political opinion softening towards surrogacy, the process remains fraught with risk for both the surrogate and the commissioning couple. It is clearly a valuable option for couples who are unable to conceive through more traditional assisted conception techniques, and the artificial insemination of the surrogate is a relatively straightforward procedure. However, the arrangement risks viewing a child as a commodity to be sold or given away, and it distorts the concept of the family by the introduction of the surrogate. What happens if the surrogate changes her mind? What if the commissioning couple rejects the child because it is born with a congenital disorder? Should the surrogate be able to command a fee for her services and will she demand more money if she suffers ill health during pregnancy?

CASE STUDY: Surrogate mother has twins

A surrogate who was 25 weeks' pregnant found she was carrying twins and says that the commissioning couple abandoned the surrogacy arrangement because of this (John, 2005). The arrangement called for selective reduction if the surrogate became pregnant with more than one foetus, but the commissioning couple now wanted to abandon the arrangement altogether.

A second couple then approached the surrogate and agreed to receive the babies.

CASE STUDY: *Surrogate changes her mind*

In the UK, a 31-year-old married surrogate was commissioned to have a child for a Dutch couple who had paid her £12,000 expenses three days after she became pregnant using the man's sperm (Watson-Smyth, 1997).

The relationship between the surrogate and the commissioning couple soured and the surrogate withdrew, determined to keep the baby and even falsely claiming that she had terminated the pregnancy.

The case studies above illustrate the complex dilemmas faced by both the commissioning couple and the surrogate. The approach of successive governments to the problem has been largely to ignore it by refusing to regulate the practice, other than to ensure that no third party or agency commercialises the process.

The Surrogacy Arrangements Act 1985 was enacted after the case of baby Cotton came to light in the UK. Baby Cotton was not the first baby to be born of a surrogate mother in Britain. The others were conceived by private arrangements between the surrogates and the childless couples. It was the use of a middleman based on a US-style commercial agency extracting large fees from desperate would-be parents that prompted accusations of exploitation and degrading the process of childbirth and motherhood. The 1985 Act outlawed commercial surrogacy and the activities that agencies would carry out, such as finding the parties and advertising for a surrogate.

The three in the party, that is, the surrogate and the commissioning couple, commit no crime, as Parliament does not want the child born to criminalised parents even if money was paid. Agencies offering assistance on a non-fee basis are lawful and health professionals who assist in a surrogacy arrangement are also generally free from prosecution.

Aside from outlawing commercial surrogacy, the government has imposed no further regulation on surrogacy arrangements and makes it clear under the provisions of section 1A of the Surrogacy Arrangements Act 1985 that *No surrogacy arrangement is enforceable by or against any of the persons making it*. There is no contract and the courts will not enforce a surrogacy arrangement. It does, therefore, make it a risky business for all the parties.

Consequences for parenthood

Under the provisions of section 33 of the Human Fertilisation and Embryology Act 2008, the woman who carries or is carrying the child and no other is the mother of the child. This applies to treatment and arrangements carried out both in and outside the UK. If a surrogate is married, her husband will be regarded as the child's father, unless he can show that he did not consent to the arrangement and the common law presumption that a husband is the father of his wife's child is rebutted (Human Fertilisation and Embryology Act 2008, s35).

Where the presumption is rebutted or the surrogate is unmarried, and the surrogate and commissioning father had sex or performed unlicensed artificial insemination, the commissioning father is father of the child.

Where a man wants to be treated as the father of a child during licensed infertility treatment, then at the time the embryo or gametes have been placed in the woman or at the time she is artificially inseminated, the couple must each have given notice of consent to him being treated as the father (Human Fertilisation and Embryology Act 2008, ss37 and 38).

Parental orders

A parental order transfers parenthood from a surrogate and her husband or partner, if she has one, to the couple who commissioned the surrogacy arrangement.

The Human Fertilisation and Embryology Act 2008 now enables same-sex couples and unmarried couples as well as married couples to apply for a parental order. This part of the Act came into force in April 2010.

Human Fertilisation and Embryology Act 1990 as amended

The Human Fertilisation and Embryology Act 1990 created a national system for the licensing and regulation for research and fertility treatment, including the storage of gametes and embryos. The process is overseen by the Human Fertilisation and Embryology Authority (HFEA), whose functions are informed by both men and women from a range of backgrounds. The chair, deputy chair and at least half of the HFEA members cannot be medical practitioners or those involved in assisted conception or its research.

The 1990 Act framed assisted conception law for heterosexual couples and aimed to promote traditional family values and the institution of marriage by discouraging same-sex and single parents. Clinics were placed under an obligation to consider a child's need for a father before offering treatment and, in practice, this meant that they were reluctant to treat single and lesbian women.

The science of fertility has advanced considerably since 1990. It is now possible to vet embryos for genetic disorders, tissue-match embryos with sick siblings, choose the sex of a child and genetically manipulate embryos. The Human Fertilisation and Embryology Act 2008 amends the 1990 Act to bring the law up to date with these scientific advances and set new ethical boundaries designed to maintain public confidence in fertility treatment. The 2008 Act prohibits sex selection for non-medical reasons and puts on a statutory footing the rules on embryo testing, research and storage.

This is done through the HFEA, which regulates the activities of the Act through a code of practice, informs the public about treatments and advances in fertility research, and reports to the Secretary of State for Health. It also grants licences to clinics and research establishments.

Licensed treatment

Fertility clinics must have a licence in order to:

- create embryos in vitro (outside the body);
- keep and store embryos;
- use donated gametes in treatment;
- test the viability of embryos;
- place a permitted embryo in woman;
- undertake tests, such as fertility tests using gametes;
- store gametes, embryos or both.

A licence is also required for research using embryos, such as the in vitro creation of embryos.

No licence will be granted unless the HFEA is satisfied that the research is necessary to:

- promote advances in infertility treatment;
- investigate causes of congenital disease;

- investigate causes of miscarriage;
- allow more effective contraception;
- detect chromosome or gene abnormality.

The often rapid advances in the science of fertility, congenital disorders and testing require the HFEA to make judgements about the ethical implications of using these discoveries in practice.

CASE STUDY: Egg donation

The HFEA wrote to all licensed clinics telling them not to practise egg giving, an arrangement whereby a person seeking IVF treatment agrees at the outset to go through one treatment cycle in which all the eggs collected are donated to a second person, followed by a further IVF cycle for their own treatment at reduced cost.

The HFEA was concerned about the extra risk of ovarian hyperstimulation syndrome (OHSS). Although this is low (at about 1 per cent), women taking part in egg giving programmes run this risk twice because they have to have two cycles of treatment (HFEA, 2003).

Consent and counselling

The law requires counselling to be offered and information to be provided before:

- treatment with donated gametes or embryos;
- treatment that will create embryos in vitro;
- storage of gametes or embryos;
- donation of gametes or embryos for the treatment of others;
- donation of gametes for use in non-medical fertility services;
- donation of embryos for research purposes;
- a person consents to be treated as the legal parent of any child born as a result of treatment.

Counselling must be a distinct service provided by the clinic and must cover implications of the treatment or donation, support counselling at times of stress, and therapeutic counselling that includes the likely success of treatment and the expectations of the parties.

Consent must be obtained for each procedure and the law requires that this consent is made in writing. The clinic must obtain written informed consent from a person before:

- storing gametes;
- using gametes for the treatment of others or for non-medical fertility services;
- creating embryos in vitro with their gametes;
- storing embryos created with their gametes;
- using embryos created with their gametes for their own treatment, treatment of a partner or treatment of others;
- using embryos created with their gametes for training people in embryo biopsy, embryo storage or other embryological techniques;
- using embryos created with their gametes for any research project;
- using their cells to create embryos for research;
- creating human admixed embryos with their gametes or cells.

The written consent to the storage of gametes or embryos must specify the storage period and state what should be done if the person giving the consent dies or loses decision-making capacity. Consent may be varied or withdrawn up to the point where the gamete or embryo is used in treatment or research.

> **CASE STUDY: Withdrawal of consent for assisted conception**
>
> In *Evans v Amicus Healthcare Ltd* [2004], two women had undergone IVF treatment with their former partners. Following the breakdown of the relationships the women still wished to have the remaining embryos implanted into them, but the men withdrew their consent.
>
> The court held that, as both couples originally sought treatment together, the embryos could not be used by just one of them. Each party had the unconditional right to withdraw consent at any time up until use, which in this context meant transfer of the embryos into the women. The withdrawal of consent was valid and assisted conception could not proceed.

Access to treatment services

No treatment services regulated by the HFEA can be provided unless account has been taken of the welfare of any child who may be born as a result, and of any other child who may be affected by the birth. Treatment centres are obliged to take reasonable steps to protect those seeking treatment and children from harm to health. This will include an assessment of the parties':

- commitment;
- ability to provide a supportive environment;
- medical and social histories;
- age and future caring ability;
- risk of harm, including:
  - abuse;
  - inherited disorders;
  - transmissible disease.

> **CASE STUDY: Refusal of treatment**
>
> In *R v Ethical Committee of St Mary's Hospital Ex p. Harriott* [1988], a woman unable to conceive a child had an application to adopt refused because of her criminal record for offences related to prostitution. She then sought an in vitro fertilisation, but was also turned down for treatment when the ethics committee became aware of the refused adoption application and the reasons for refusal. The woman challenged the decision.
>
> The court held that the committee had no duty to investigate the matter and the court would not interfere unless the committee's advice was illegal or discriminatory and, in this case, it was not.

Donors

Selection of donors for licensed treatment must be subject to the same written consent and counselling as for those seeking treatment. A potential donor must be screened and assessed to determine if they have a particular gene, chromosome or mitochondrial abnormality that, if inherited, may result in that child having or developing serious physical or mental disability, serious illness or any other serious medical condition. Children born with such an illness or disability may seek redress through the courts under the Congenital Disability (Civil Liability) Act 1976.

The donor of sperm or an egg donor cannot be treated as the parent of any child resulting from the use of their gametes in the licensed treatment of others. The identity of donors was generally kept confidential, but donor conception is becoming less secretive. The Human Fertilisation and Embryology Act 2008 amends the information rights available in connection with donor conception and gives new rights to donor-conceived people to contact their genetic siblings. Donor anonymity was lifted in 2005, allowing children conceived after this date to obtain identifying information about their donors when they become 18.

Private insemination arrangements are more common, as it is relatively simple and there is no law against do-it-yourself insemination. However, the law determining who are the legal parents of the child is strict and cannot be overridden. For same-sex couples, paternity depends on whether or not the arrangement meets the conditions of section 42 of the 2008 Act, which are:

- the mother was inseminated artificially;
- the insemination occurred on or after 6 April 2009;
- the mother was in a civil partnership at the time of the insemination;
- the mother's civil partner consented to the insemination.

If it does, the mother's civil partner will be the child's second parent and the biological father has no legal connection with the child. If it does not, then the sperm donor is the father.

For heterosexual couples the conditions are:

- the mother was inseminated artificially;
- the mother was married at the time of the insemination;
- the mother's husband consented to the insemination.

If the arrangement does not fall into these conditions, the sperm donor counts as the father and:

- the mother could seek child maintenance from the donor;
- the father could seek contact with the child even if the mother does not agree;
- if the mother wants a future partner to be the child's other parent, the biological father would have to agree to an adoption or the court overrule the father's objection.

Recognition of dead partners

A husband or male partner who has provided sperm for the treatment of their wife or female partner can be registered as the father of a child born as a result of treatment after their death, if:

- the man had given written consent for his sperm, or embryos created using his sperm, to be used after his death in the treatment of his wife or partner;
- the man had given written consent to being registered as the father of any resulting child;

- the woman elected in writing, within 42 days after the child's birth (21 days in Scotland), for the man's details to be entered in the relevant register of births;
- no one else is to be treated as the father or parent of the child.

A partner (husband, civil partner or other partner) who has not provided sperm for the treatment of their wife or female partner can be registered as the father or parent of any child born as a result of treatment after their death, if:

- the treatment involved the transfer to the woman of an embryo after the death of the partner;
- the embryo was created when the partner was alive;
- the partner had given written consent for the embryo to be placed in the woman after his death;
- the partner had given written consent to being registered as the father or parent of any resulting child;
- the woman elected in writing, within 42 days after the child's birth (21 days in Scotland), for the partner's details to be entered in the relevant register of births;
- no one else is to be treated as the father or parent of the child.

Conscientious objection to participation in abortion and assisted conception techniques

The Abortion Act 1967, section 4, and the Human Fertilisation and Embryology Act 1990 both allow conscientious objection to participating in such treatment, other than where the treatment is necessary to save the life of the mother. The objection must be made ahead of any treatment and it is for health professionals to prove the conscientious objection if they rely on it as a defence in any legal proceedings. The objection only applies to treatment, not to other related activity.

CASE STUDY: What constitutes treatment?

In *Janaway v Salford HA* [1988], a medical secretary lost her appeal against her dismissal for refusing to type a letter referring a patient for a termination of pregnancy. The House of Lords held that participation in treatment meant to take part in treatment for the purpose of terminating a pregnancy. Simply typing a letter of referral could not be regarded as taking part in the treatment and she was not entitled to refuse to do so.

C   H   A   P   T   E   R   S   U   M   M   A   R   Y

- Abortion is any treatment to terminate a pregnancy. To be lawful, a termination of pregnancy must be covered by the provisions of the Abortion Act 1967.
- Procuring a miscarriage is an offence under the Offences Against the Person Act 1861. The Infant Life (Preservation) Act 1929 makes it an offence to kill a child capable of being born alive before it had an existence independent of its mother.
- The use of the morning-after pill is not abortion.

- Under English law an unborn child has no legal rights until it is born alive, therefore any conflict of interest between the mother and the foetus is resolved in favour of the mother.
- It is an offence for a mother or any person present at the birth, including the midwife, to conceal the birth of a child.
- There is a legal duty on the midwife attending a woman in labour to notify the PCT for the area of the birth and whether the baby was born alive or dead. It is the duty of the baby's father or mother to register the birth.
- A baby born at any stage of pregnancy who breathes or shows other signs of life after complete expulsion from its mother is born alive.
- A stillborn child is a child born after the twenty-fourth week of pregnancy who did not at any time after being completely delivered from its mother breathe or show any other signs of life.
- Surrogacy is a practice whereby one woman carries a child for another with the intention that the child should be handed over at birth. The woman who carries the child, and no other, is the mother of the child.
- A parental order transfers parenthood from a surrogate and her husband or partner to the couple who commissioned the surrogacy.
- The Human Fertilisation and Embryology Act 1990 created a national system for the regulation of fertility treatment.
- The Abortion Act 1967 and the Human Fertilisation and Embryology Act 1990 both allow a conscientious objection to participating in treatment other than where necessary to save the life of the mother.

Knowledge review

Having completed the chapter, how would you now rate your knowledge of the following topics?

	Good	Adequate	Poor
1. The law relating to the termination of pregnancy.			
2. The rights bestowed on an unborn child.			
3. Surrogacy, and how it is regulated in the UK.			
4. The regulation of assisted conception by the Human Fertilisation and Embryology Act 1990 (as amended).			

Where you're not confident in your knowledge of a topic, what will you do next?

Further reading

Jackson, E (2001) *Regulating Reproduction: Law, technology and autonomy.* London: Hart Publishing.
Gives an in-depth consideration of the law and reproduction.

Mason, JK (2007) *The Troubled Pregnancy: Legal wrongs and rights in reproduction.*
Cambridge: Cambridge University Press.
Examines the ethics of regulating pregnancy and reproduction.

Useful websites

www.brook.org.uk Brook, which is a national voluntary sector provider of free and confidential sexual health advice and services specifically for young people under 25.
www.hfea.gov.uk Human Fertilisation and Embryology Authority, which gives a comprehensive guide to the implementation of the Human Fertilisation and Embryology Acts.

Chapter 13

Medicines and the law

Chapter aims

After reading this chapter, you will be able to:

- state the principle sources of law governing the safety of medicines;
- outline the three classifications of medicines used in the UK;
- describe the alternatives to prescription for the supply and administration of prescription-only medicines by midwives;
- discuss the value to practice of midwives becoming non-medical prescribers;
- explain the legal requirements for the possession and use of controlled drugs in midwifery practice.

Introduction

Medicines are used for their curative benefits and make an important contribution to the therapeutic interventions used in healthcare. Some 7,000 doses of medication are administered each day in an average general hospital. In the community, five million consultations with GPs, nurses and midwives result in ten million medicines being dispensed by pharmacists each week. They are a vital therapeutic weapon in the health service's armoury.

As well as their beneficial effects, medicines also have great potential to harm those who take them and this risk increases in pregnant women and babies. Some 10,000 serious adverse drug reactions are reported each year in the UK. The European Commission reports that 5 per cent of hospital admissions are due to the adverse effects of medicines and that they are the fifth most common cause of death in hospital.

This chapter will consider the laws relating to medicines that have been established to protect the public, and their specific relevance to midwifery practice. First of all, it will consider further why such laws are needed. It will then examine the sources of these laws, before looking at the laws themselves.

The need for medicine laws in midwifery practice

> **CASE STUDY: The thalidomide case**
>
> Thalidomide was a drug that was marketed as a sedative with apparently remarkably few side effects. It was believed to be so safe that it could be prescribed to pregnant women to help combat morning sickness. Drug testing procedures and the reporting of adverse drug reactions were far more relaxed in the 1950s and 1960s. Tests had taken place on thalidomide but did not reveal any of its teratogenic properties (the causing of birth defects) because the tests were conducted on rodents, which metabolised the drug in a different way from humans. Later tests on rabbits and monkeys produced the same horrific side effects as in humans.
>
> The most renowned adverse effect is phocomelia, the flipper-like limbs that appeared on the children of women who took thalidomide. In the UK, the drug was licensed in 1958 and, of the 2,000 babies born with defects, 456 survived. The drug was withdrawn in 1961, but it was not until 1968, following a long campaign by the *Sunday Times* Insight team, that a compensation settlement for the UK victims was reached with pharmaceutical company Distillers Limited (*S v Distillers Co (Biochemicals)* (1969)).

This case demonstrates why it is so important to have regulation concerning medicines. The thalidomide case ultimately prompted Parliament to introduce the Medicines Act 1968, which strengthened the requirements for testing, licensing and supplying medicines to the public.

Simply put, the purpose of using the law to regulate the marketing, supply and administration of medicines is to ensure that:

- *the right medicine* is given to
- *the right person* at
- *the right time* in
- *the right form* and at
- *the right dose.*

The five Rs are particularly, and frighteningly, pertinent when working with children and babies, as is clear from the situations described below.

Scenarios

The decimal point error

A one-day-old baby died when she received a morphine dose 100 times the intended amount in hospital. An error in calculating the correct dose of the drug for the neonate resulted in the decimal point being put in the wrong place, and within two hours of being given the drug the baby was dead.

Failing to check a syringe label

A neonate died when she received a whole day's dose of morphine in 11 minutes because no one checked the label of the syringe before giving the drug. The baby was given the drug that had been prepared for an older and heavier baby.

The Medicines Act 1968 and its regulations form one strand of a series of laws that come together to provide maximum protection to the public from the harmful effects of medicines. The next sections will examine the sources of these laws and the relevant laws for midwifery practice.

Sources of medicines law

Laws relating to medicines originate from a variety of sources, including EU law, public law, common law and professional regulation.

European Union law

As we saw in our consideration of the legal system in Chapter 1, EU law is an increasingly important source of law in the UK. In common with most developments in health and safety law, recent advances in legal regulation of the safety of medicines are largely done on a Europe-wide basis. This is normally achieved by the EU issuing a directive to member states to introduce laws according to their instructions. The EU's influence on the laws that govern the safety of medicines includes:

- the criteria for deciding which medicines should be prescription only (Council Directive 92/26/EEC);
- requiring Braille labelling of the outer packaging of medicines (European Parliament and Council Directive 2004/27/EC);
- the requirements for conducting clinical trials (Council Directive 2001/20/EC).

Public law

Public law is the source of a variety of important laws relating to medicines, including the Medicines Act 1968 mentioned above. This Act controls the marketing, supply and administration of medicines to the public. Other important laws include:

- **Misuse of Drugs Act 1971** and the **Misuse of Drugs Regulations 2001**, which regulate the supply and administration of medicines that may be misused because of their addictive qualities;
- **Consumer Protection Act 1987**, which gives statutory protection to the public from harmful products, making the manufacturer strictly liable for harm caused by a defective product, including medicines.

We will look at these in more detail later in the chapter.

Common law

Common law also has established some key laws in this area, including the following.

- Trespass law (see Chapters 5 and 6). This ensures that medicines are only administered with the consent of a person with capacity or in the best interests of a person who lacks decision-making capacity. Even where a midwife is a prescriber, or is acting on the instruction of a prescriber or other exemption under the Medicines Act 1968, this does not do away with the need for consent before administering the medicine.
- The law of negligence (see Chapter 10). This imposes a legal duty on midwives to take care when supplying or administering medicines. Any harm to a mother or baby that results from a midwife's carelessness in selecting, supplying, administering or calculating the dose of a drug will result in the midwife being liable in negligence. Where the grossly negligent actions of the midwife result in the death of a woman, the midwife could face prosecution for manslaughter.

Professional regulation

Finally, the midwives' professional regulatory body, the NMC, imposes standards on midwifery practice through the Nursing and Midwifery Order 2001, the *Midwives Rules and Standards* (2004b) and *The Code* (2008a). In the case of medicines, the NMC also sets out 26 *Standards for Medicines Management* (2008c). Midwives are held to account for their medicines management against these standards and a midwife who falls below the standard required can face charges of professional misconduct at a fitness to practise hearing (see Chapter 3). We will look at these professional requirements in relation to medicines in more detail later in the chapter.

The legal regulation of medicines

Here, we will look in more detail at some of the most important laws that you will need to be familiar with.

Consumer Protection Act 1987

Initial statutory protection for all products is given by the Consumer Protection Act 1987, which protects consumers from harmful products, including medicines. Strict liability (or liability without fault) makes a producer liable for damage caused by an inherently defective product (Council Directive 85/374/EEC, article 8(2)).

Where a person is harmed by an inherent defect in a medicine, it will be the producer *not* the midwife who will be liable, as can be seen from the case below.

CASE STUDY: The digestible sponge case

In *Les Laboratoires Leo SA v Scovazzo* [1999], a medicines manufacturer developed a drug with a digestible sponge coating designed to delay absorption of the drug until it reached the lower intestine.

The use of the digestible sponge coating was less than successful and it caused severe inflammation of the intestine in many patients. The manufacturer was held strictly liable for the harm caused.

Medicines Act 1968

The principal statute regulating the use of medicines is the Medicines Act 1968. This provides an administrative and licensing system to control the sale and supply of medicines to the public. Generally, before a drug can be marketed for sale or supply to the public it must have a product licence or marketing authorisation issued by the Secretary of State for Health. The licence is not published, but its provisions are summarised in the data sheet issued with the medicine and available in the *Association of the British Pharmaceutical Industry Data Sheet Compendium*, published annually in January. It is essential that all student midwives are aware of, and comply with, the licensed uses of the most common medicinal products used in midwifery practice.

Activity 13.1	Evidence-based practice and research

- Visit the electronic medicines compendium that contains the data sheet of all licensed medicines in the UK at **http://emc.medicines.org.uk**.
- Search for some of the medicines you have used in practice and note their licensed uses and main adverse reactions.

As this activity will be based on your own research, there is no outline answer at the end of the chapter.

A product licence or marketing authorisation cannot be issued unless the Commission on Human Medicines, under the supervision of the Medicines and Healthcare products Regulatory Agency (MHRA), has been consulted (Medicines Act 1968, s2). This body is charged with looking at matters such as the quality of the drug and its usefulness for the purpose for which it is promoted. The MHRA is further charged with the collection of data on adverse reactions to the drug (Medicines Act 1968, s4).

Classification of drugs

Activity 13.2	Evidence-based practice and research

Before moving on, list the types of medicines and pack sizes you have seen for sale or being supplied in the following places:

- on the shelves of a fuel station, shop or supermarket;
- in a community pharmacy or store with a pharmacy.

You may wish to visit a shop or a pharmacy to create a more comprehensive list.

As this activity will be based on your own research, there is no outline answer at the end of the chapter.

Drugs that have a product licence or marketing authorisation are categorised into three types for the purpose of supply to the general public: general sales list drugs, pharmacy-only drugs and drugs that can only be bought with a prescription.

General sales list drugs

This type of drug may be sold through a variety of outlets without need for a registered pharmacist. They contain ingredients that can be sold from any lockable shop. Typically, the main outlets for these are grocery stores, health food shops and petrol station shops. People can select the medicine off the shelf. The general sales list includes small packs of analgesics containing aspirin, paracetamol and ibuprofen, most antacids, simple cough mixtures, throat pastilles and antiseptics.

Pharmacy-only drugs

This category of medicine can only be purchased under the supervision of a registered pharmacist in a retail pharmacy. The packaging of the medicine is marked with a 'P'. Products include medicines recently removed from prescription control. They may have restrictions on age of patients, indications, pack size and duration of treatment compared with their use on prescription. Self-selection of these medicines is not allowed, so they can only be supplied from behind the counter in pharmacies. Examples include ranitidine (for heartburn in pregnancy), cimetidine (to control gastric acid reflux) and piriton (for allergies, especially the relief of hay fever, and safer than alternatives when pregnant).

Prescription-only drugs

The Medicines Act 1968, section 58A, requires that medicines that represent a danger to the public be classified as prescription only and their administration be supervised by an appropriate practitioner. This category of medicine can only be obtained from a registered pharmacist by prescription from an appropriate practitioner, such as registered doctor, dentist or non-medical prescriber (Medicines Act 1968, s58). They include relatively new medicines, medicines that require medical monitoring of effectiveness or adverse effects, and medicines that are frequently used incorrectly. All medicines that are for injection are also prescription only.

Prescription-only medicines cannot be promoted or advertised to the public. They cannot normally be supplied unless a prescription has been issued from an appropriate practitioner. In exceptional circumstances, pharmacists may supply five days' emergency treatment of a prescription-only product (Medicines (Products Other Than Veterinary Drugs) (Prescription Only) Order 1983).

The criteria for determining which products should be available on prescription only are regulated by Directive 92/26/EEC. These medicines are listed in article 3 of the Prescription Only Medicines (Human Use) Order 1997.

Appropriate practitioners

In addition to regulating how a drug can be marketed for sale or supplied to the public, the Medicines Act 1968 also regulates who can prescribe prescription-only drugs. Section 58(1) of the Act bestows prescribing authority on registered medical practitioners and dentists, who are therefore able to issue prescriptions for medicines. The Medicinal Products: Prescribing by Nurses etc. Act 1992 and the Health & Social Care Act 2001, section 63, extended the range of professionals who can act as appropriate practitioners. The Medicines for Human Use (Prescribing) (Miscellaneous Amendments) Order 2006 introduced three categories of non-medical prescriber:

- independent prescriber;
- independent/supplementary prescriber;
- community practitioner prescriber.

Under the 2006 regulations, registered midwives whose names are held on the NMC professional register, with an annotation signifying that they have successfully completed an approved programme of preparation and training, can be independent and/or supplementary prescribers.

Prescriptions

There are also specific laws relating to what is classified as a prescription. Under the National Health Service Act 1977, a prescription is an instruction issued by an appropriate practitioner to supply a prescription-only medicine to a patient – that is, it is written on the proscribed form and is signed and dated by the practitioner.

Article 15 of the Prescription Only Medicines (Human Use) Order 1997 requires that a prescription must be completed and signed in ink, or be otherwise indelible (a large number of prescriptions are now computer-generated), on the statutory form and must contain the following information:

- the name and address of the patient;
- the drug and dose described clearly;
- the signature of the prescriber;
- the date of signing;
- the address of the appropriate practitioner;
- the status of the appropriate practitioner (e.g. midwife independent prescriber).

Definitions

It is vital that student midwives understand the key terms used in medicines management, some of which have specific legal definitions.

Activity 13.3   *Reflection*

Before moving on, write down what you understand the following terms to mean:

- administration of a medicine;
- parenteral administration of a medicine;
- supply;
- manufacture.

Please do not move on to the next part until you are ready for the answer.

Administration

The term 'administration' does not have a definition set out in law. It is accepted as involving the medicine being given by the midwife or the midwife supervising the mother taking the dose.

Parenteral administration

The Prescription Only Medicines (Human Use) Order 1997 defines 'parenteral administration' as administration by breach of the skin or mucous membrane. This would include the midwife giving a subcutaneous or intramuscular injection.

Supply

The Medicines Act 1968, section 131, defines 'supply' as supplying a drug in circumstances corresponding to retail sale. This would occur where midwives were providing any medicine for the mothers in their care to take away and administer themselves. For example, a midwife supplying a medicine under a patient group direction (PGD) (see pages 224–6) must issue the medicine in a prepacked form suitable for the woman to take away. The midwife cannot issue a note for the mother to take to a pharmacist to supply the medicine.

Manufacture

The Medicines Act 1968, section 132, defines 'manufacture' in relation to a medicine as any process carried out in the course of making the product.

It therefore does not include dissolving or dispersing the product in water, or diluting or mixing it with some other substance used for the purpose of administering it.

This definition of manufacture means that a tablet can be crushed or a capsule opened and mixed with a solution to make it easier for a person to swallow, although the midwife must ensure that there is sound evidence that this is safe to do. The definition also allows midwives to mix powdered medicines with, for example, water prior to injection.

However, mixing two medicines falls within the definition of manufacture and a new unlicensed product would be created.

Midwives cannot supply or administer an unlicensed medicine unless they are independent or supplementary prescribers or have been instructed by a doctor. They cannot mix two medicines unless this has been sanctioned by the prescriber and is shown by the available evidence to be safe.

Administration of medicines

A drug categorised as a prescription-only medicine can normally only be administered by, or under the direction of, the prescriber, who is referred to as the appropriate practitioner. The Medicines Act 1968, section 58(2)(b), states that:

> No person shall administer otherwise than to himself any such medicinal product unless he is an appropriate practitioner or a person acting in accordance with the directions of an appropriate practitioner.

As a general rule, midwives supplying or administering a prescription-only medicine will need to do so in accordance with the instructions of the prescriber. However, to overcome the need to send a mother to a doctor each time she needed a prescription, or to a pharmacy to obtain medicines, a range of exemptions remove registered midwives from the general rules regulating the supply and administration of medicines under the Medicines Act 1968.

Exemption from restriction on supply of medicines

Under the provisions of the Medicines (Pharmacy and General Sale – Exemption) Order 1980, article 4, and Medicines (Sale or Supply) (Miscellaneous Provisions) Regulations 1980, registered midwives may supply, but not sell, during the course of their practice all medicines categorised as general sales list and pharmacy-only medicines. Midwives can therefore supply the wide range of medicines available on these lists as long as it is appropriate for the needs of the mother or baby and is done during the course of the midwife's practice. As we have seen, supply means issuing a medicine in circumstances corresponding to retail sale. The midwife must therefore supply the medicine in a package suitable for the woman to take away and administer herself. The midwife cannot use these exemptions to issue an instruction to a pharmacist to dispense and supply the medicine.

Midwives can also supply a limited range of prescription-only medicines in an exemption set out in the Prescription Only Medicines (Human Use) Order 1997, schedule 5. This sets out the medicines that can be supplied and the conditions that must be met before the midwife is entitled to supply them, as described in Table 13.1.

The medicine in square brackets in Table 13.1 was added by the Prescription Only Medicines (Human Use) Amendment (No. 3) Order 1998.

Although the Prescription Only Medicines (Human Use) Order 1997 gives registered midwives exemption from restriction on supply for a number of prescription-only medicines, it also highlights the limitation of such exemptions, which are inflexible and cannot easily be changed to reflect developments in practice. Most of the medicines in the exempt list are no longer considered to be medicines of choice in current midwifery practice and oral ergometrine is no longer available in the British National Formulary (Jordan, 2009). The MHRA (2008) consulted on proposals to update the list of medicines contained in the midwives' exemption list in 2008, but no amendments have been made to date.

Exemption from restrictions on administration of prescription-only medicines

In addition to the relatively broad exemption for the supply of medicines to mothers during the course of their practice, midwives also have a limited exemption to administer, without prescription, a number of prescription-only medicines under the provisions of the Prescription Only Medicines (Human Use) Order 1997, schedule 5, article 11(2).

The medicines in square brackets in Table 13.2 were added by the Prescription Only Medicines (Human Use) Amendment Order 2004.

The exemption only applies to the parenteral administration of the medicine in the course of a midwife's professional practice and in the case of promazine and lignocaine only when attending a woman in childbirth. Provided the requirements of any conditions

Table 13.1: Prescription Only Medicines (Human Use) Order 1997, schedule 5: Exemption from restrictions on sale or supply

Persons exempted	Prescription-only medicines to which the exemption applies	Conditions
Registered midwives.	Prescription-only medicines containing any of the following substances: • chloral hydrate • ergometrine maleate • pentazocine hydrochloride • [phytomenadione] • triclofos sodium.	The sale or supply shall be only in the course of their professional practice and in the case of ergometrine maleate only when contained in a medicinal product that is not for parenteral administration.

Table 13.2: Prescription Only Medicines (Human Use) Order 1997, schedule 5: Exemption from restrictions on administration

Persons exempted	Prescription-only medicines to which the exemption applies	Conditions
Registered midwives.	Prescription-only medicines for parenteral administration containing any of the following substances but no other substance specified in column 1 of schedule 1 to this Order: • [diamorphine] • ergometrine maleate • lignocaine • lignocaine hydrochloride • [morphine] • naloxone hydrochloride • oxytocins, natural and synthetic • pentazocine lactate • pethidine hydrochloride • phytomenadione • promazine hydrochloride.	The administration shall be only in the course of their professional practice and in the case of promazine hydrochloride, lignocaine and lignocaine hydrochloride shall be only while attending a woman in childbirth.

attached to the exemptions are met, there is no need for a prescription or PGD for that medicine.

Exemption for the administration of a prescription-only medicine in an emergency

In addition to the specific exemptions for midwives, a general exemption on restriction from parenteral administration is allowed for medicinal products for the purpose of saving life in an emergency (Prescription Only Medicines (Human Use) Order 1997, article 7). There is no specific restriction on who is entitled to administer these medicines, so a midwife may administer these medicines where appropriate to save life in an emergency:

• adrenaline injection 1 in 1000 (1 mg in 1 ml);
• [atropine sulphate and obidoxime chloride injection];
• [atropine sulphate and pralidoxime chloride injection];
• atropine sulphate injection;
• [atropine sulphate, pralidoxime mesilate and avizafone injection];
• [chlorphenamine injection];
• [dicobalt edetate injection];
• glucagon injection;
• [glucose injection 50%];
• hydrocortisone injection;
• [naloxone hydrochloride];
• [pralidoxime chloride injection];
• [pralidoxime mesilate injection];

- promethazine hydrochloride injection;
- snake venom antiserum;
- sodium nitrite injection;
- sodium thiosulphate injection;
- sterile pralidoxime.

The medicines in square brackets were added later by the Prescription Only Medicines (Human Use) Amendment (No. 3) Order 2004. It should be noted that pralidoxime mesilate and avizafone injection are not in the British National Formulary (BNF). A practical use for the exemptions is demonstrated in the scenario below.

Scenario

At a midwife-led antenatal clinic, around ten expectant mothers attend each session. Although they are low risk, several of them have pregnancy-related conditions. There is no doctor present at the clinic, but the midwife is able to supply a range of medicines for the mothers' conditions as they are medicines that are categorised as general sales list or pharmacy medicines.

The midwife can supply these medicines without the need for a prescription under the exemption from restriction on supply in the Medicines (Pharmacy and General Sale – Exemption) Order 1980, article 4, and Medicines (Sale or Supply) (Miscellaneous Provisions) Regulations 1980.

It would therefore be possible for the midwife in the course of her practice to supply the following, in a form suitable to be taken away and self-administered:

- ranitidine hydrochloride, a pharmacy medicine, to a woman who complained of acid indigestion;
- ferrous sulphate, a pharmacy medicine, to a woman who had iron-deficiency anaemia;
- lactulose, a pharmacy medicine, to a woman suffering from constipation;
- Anusol Plus HC® ointment, a general sales list medicine, to a woman with haemorrhoids.

Midwifery Standing Orders

The NMC has acknowledged that, in the past, maternity service providers have extended the range of medicines used by midwives without prescription by producing local guidelines, often referred to as Standing Orders, to supplement the exemptions from restriction on supply and administration of medicines. These guidelines are not sanctioned under any legislation and there is no legal definition of Standing Orders, as the term does not exist in any of the medicines legislation.

The NMC now requires that all maternity services restrict the supply and administration of medicines by midwives without prescription to those covered by the exemptions to the Medicines Act 1968 contained in the Prescription Only Medicines (Human Use) Order 1997. Any Standing Orders for medicines outside those exemptions must now be converted to Patient Group Directions (NMC, 2008c).

Patient group directions

A patient group direction (PGD) is a written instruction for the supply or administration of a licensed medicine in an identified clinical situation where the patient may not be individually identified before presenting for treatment. It allows a midwife to supply or administer a prescription-only medicine to a woman without prescription if she meets the conditions set out in the PGD.

A PGD must be drawn up locally by doctors, pharmacists and midwives and must meet legal criteria set out in the Prescription Only Medicines (Human Use) Amendment Order 2000.

Concept summary: Legal requirements for a valid PGD

- The name of the body to which the direction applies.
- The date the direction comes into force and the date it expires.
- A description of the medicine(s) to which the direction applies.
- The clinical conditions covered by the direction.
- A description of those patients excluded from treatment under the direction.
- A description of the circumstances under which further advice should be sought from a doctor (or dentist, as appropriate) and arrangements for referral made.
- Appropriate dosage and maximum total dosage, quantity, pharmaceutical form and strength, route and frequency of administration, and minimum or maximum period over which the medicine should be administered.
- Relevant warnings, including potential adverse reactions.
- Details of any follow-up action and the circumstances.
- A statement of the records to be kept for audit purposes.
- Names and signatures of registered practitioners entitled to supply and/or administer medicines under the PGD.

PGDs are intended for local use. Each one must be signed by a senior doctor and a senior pharmacist, and approved by the organisation in which it is to be used, typically a PCT or Local Health Board.

PGDs can only be used by registered healthcare professionals, including midwives, and a list of individuals named as competent to supply and administer medicines under the direction must be included. The NMC (2009b) has made it clear that student midwives cannot supply or administer medicines using a PGD.

PGDs can include a flexible dose range for the midwife to select from for the mother or baby. Medicines can also be used off-licence, or off-label (see page 000), provided such use is supported by best clinical practice and the PGD contains a statement as to why this is necessary.

PGDs and controlled drugs

The Misuse of Drugs Regulations 2001 now allow some controlled drugs to be supplied and/or administered under a PGD. These include all drugs listed in Schedule 4 of the 2001 Regulations (mostly benzodiazepines), except anabolic steroids and all drugs listed in schedule 5 of the 2001 Regulations (these are mainly low-strength opiates such as codeine).

The National Prescribing Centre (2004) suggests that the supply and administration of medicines under PGDs should be reserved for the limited number of situations where this offers an advantage for the care of individuals without compromising safety. It further suggests that particular caution should be used when deciding whether to use a PGD for an antibiotic, as antimicrobial resistance is a public health issue of great concern and care should be taken to ensure that any strategy to control increasing resistance will not be jeopardised. For example, a PGD should not allow the supply or administration of a medicine for minor viral diseases that are unaffected by antibiotics, such as sore throats, in the absence of good evidence of bacterial infection. However, as the scenario below illustrates, allowing the supply of antibiotics in clearly defined cases will allow midwives to provide timely treatment to mothers.

Scenario

An expectant mother attends a midwife-led antenatal clinic at her local health centre, where she is told that she has an uncomplicated genital infection caused by chlamydia.

Erythromicin is the drug of choice for this condition but, as a prescription-only medicine, it cannot usually be supplied without a prescription. However, a PGD is in place that allows the midwife to supply the drug to the woman without prescription as the criteria set out in the direction have been met.

The midwife supplies the woman with the erythromycin in a take-home pack, giving her clear instructions for its administration and a further clinic appointment in five weeks to test whether the medicine has cured the infection.

Patient specific direction

A patient specific direction (PSD) is a written instruction for medicines to be supplied for administering to a named patient. The most common use of a PSD is the instruction to administer medicines written on a hospital ward drug administration chart. A PSD differs from a prescription. To be lawful, a prescription must meet the requirements of article 15 of the Prescription Only Medicines (Human Use) Order 1997 (see page 219). A PSD is lawful even if it does not meet these requirements, and a midwife is entitled to administer medicines in accordance with a PSD.

As a PSD is individually tailored to the needs of a single person, it should be used in preference to a PGD where possible. Article 12 of the Prescription Only Medicines (Human Use) Order 1997, which authorises the use of PSDs, allows any appropriate practitioner (including midwives with independent prescribing authority) to write a written instruction for the supply and administration of a prescription-only medicine in a hospital.

Article 12A of the 1997 Order allows for the use of a PSD in the community by giving an exemption for the supply and administration of prescription-only medicines by an NHS body. This applies where the medicine is supplied for the purpose of being administered to a particular person in accordance with the written directions of a doctor, even though the direction does not satisfy the conditions for a valid prescription. So a GP could authorise a midwife to administer a prescription-only medicine to a mother in her care by making an entry in the woman's medical record.

The Medicines Act 1968 and its regulations provide midwives with a degree of flexibility with regard to the supply and administration of prescription-only medicines. As well as administering medicines according to a prescription, midwives can also supply and administer medicines through a PGD, a PSD and using midwife-specific exemptions. A further, more comprehensive, means of supplying prescription-only medicines is now available to midwives. They can become independent or supplementary prescribers who are entitled by law to issue prescriptions for prescription-only medicines.

The midwife as prescriber

The NHS (Miscellaneous Amendments Relating to Independent Prescribing) Regulations 2006 introduced independent prescribing and extended the range of medicines that non-medical prescribers can prescribe. A non-medical prescriber is any health professional who is not a doctor (e.g. a midwife, nurse or pharmacist). The regulations allow midwives who are prescribers to prescribe any medicine, other than certain controlled drugs. They can also issue private prescriptions for any medical condition they are competent to treat. As 'appropriate practitioners' for the purposes of the Medicines Act 1968, section 58(2), midwives who are independent prescribers can also give directions for the administration of any medicine they are legally allowed to prescribe, as long as they are satisfied that the person to whom they give the instructions is competent to administer the medicine.

All registered midwives can train to be independent prescribers. However, the NMC *Standards of Proficiency for Nurse and Midwife Prescribers* (NMC, 2006) state that they must have at least three years' post-registration experience before undertaking the course. Midwives who successfully complete the programme must register their prescribing qualification with the NMC before they can start prescribing.

Scenario

A community midwife visits an expectant mother in her home after she complains of fever and painful micturation. A urinalysis indicates a probable urinary tract infection.

Antibiotics are prescription-only medicines and are excluded from the midwives' exemptions. They are also not available to be supplied via a PGD, in order to limit the possibility of bacterial resistance to antibiotics.

However, the midwife is an independent non-medical prescriber and issues the mother with a prescription for a broad-spectrum antibiotic and takes a urine sample for laboratory analysis. The test result confirms that there is a bacterial infection that is susceptible to the prescribed antibiotic. The woman makes a speedy recovery with no complications.

Borderline substances, unlicensed medicines and off-label use of medicines

Borderline substances are mainly foodstuffs, such as enteral feeds and foods that are specially formulated for people with medical conditions. They also include some toiletries, such as sunblocks. Independent prescribers are able to prescribe these products, but should limit their prescriptions to the substances on the Advisory Committee on Borderline Substances approved list, which is published as Part XV of the Drug Tariff and which can also be found in the British National Formulary.

The term off-label, or off-licence, describes the use of licensed medicines in a dose, or for an age group, or by a route not in the product specification. For example, many medicines are not licensed for use with babies or pregnant women, but are used off-label because there is strong evidence of their safety and efficacy with these groups.

Midwives who are independent prescribers can prescribe off-label but, in doing so, take full responsibility for their prescribing. They will be accountable for harm caused by off label prescribing or administration.

Some medicines do not have a product licence because they are specially prepared by a pharmacist as an extemporaneous medicine, or two licensed medicines are mixed together to facilitate administration. The law also allows the manufacture and supply of unlicensed medicinal products, commonly known as specials, by pharmaceutical companies that hold a specials licence. The medicines are formulated in accordance with the requirements of a prescriber and the product must meet the special needs of the person on the prescriber's direct responsibility.

Scenario

A woman whose diabetes was controlled with metformin before she was pregnant is having difficulty continuing to take the tablets as prescribed as they make her nauseous and she often vomits. The midwife, in consultation with the woman and her GP, feels that a liquid alternative might overcome the swallowing difficulty and prescribes the drug as a liquid special medicine that can be obtained from her community pharmacist.

Supplementary prescribing

Supplementary prescribing is a voluntary prescribing partnership between the independent prescriber, who must be a doctor, and the supplementary prescriber. A supplementary prescriber can be a midwife, nurse or pharmacist (as part of their independent prescribing training) or optometrists, physiotherapists, podiatrists and radiographers (NMC, 2006).

The Prescription Only Medicines (Human Use) Order 1997 requires that, to be lawful, supplementary prescribing by a registered midwife must only occur where:

- the independent prescriber is a doctor;
- the supplementary prescriber is a registered midwife whose name is recorded in the relevant register, an annotation signifying that they are qualified to order drugs, medicines and appliances as a supplementary prescriber;
- there is a written clinical management plan relating to a named patient and to that patient's specific conditions;
- agreement to the plan is recorded by both the independent prescriber and the supplementary prescriber before it begins;
- the independent prescriber and the supplementary prescriber share access to, consult and use the same common patient record.

Following diagnosis by the doctor and agreement of the clinical management plan, the supplementary prescriber may prescribe any medicine for the patient that is referred to in the plan until the next review. There is no formulary for supplementary prescribing and no restrictions on the medical conditions that can be managed under these arrangements. The scope of supplementary prescribing is very broad and any prescription-only medicine, pharmacy medicine, general sales list medicine or controlled drug (whether licensed or unlicensed) can be issued as long as it is part of the agreed clinical management plan.

Under the Prescription Only Medicines (Human Use) Order 1997, to be lawful a clinical management plan must contain:

- the name of the patient to whom the plan relates;
- the illnesses or conditions that may be treated by the supplementary prescriber;

- the date on which the plan is to take effect and when it is to be reviewed by the doctor or dentist who is a party to the plan;
- reference to the class or description of the medicinal product that may be prescribed or administered under the plan;
- any restrictions or limitations as to the strength or dose of any product that may be prescribed or administered under the plan, and any period of administration or use of any medicinal product that may be prescribed or administered under the plan;
- relevant warnings about the known sensitivities of the patient to, or known difficulties of the patient with, particular medicinal products;
- the arrangements for notification of:
  - suspected or known adverse reactions to any medicinal product that may be prescribed or administered under the plan;
  - suspected or known adverse reactions to any other medicinal product taken at the same time as any medicinal product prescribed or administered under the plan;
  - the circumstances in which the supplementary prescriber should refer to, or seek the advice of, the doctor or dentist who is a party to the plan.

A supplementary prescriber who issues a prescription in contravention of the regulations could face prosecution and a misconduct charge from the NMC, as well as disciplinary proceedings by their employer.

Prescribing controlled drugs

Controlled drugs are prescription-only medicines that are further regulated by the Misuse of Drugs Act 1971 because of their addictive properties. Supply and possession of these drugs without prescription is generally a serious criminal offence. Many controlled drugs are used in midwifery practice, mainly for the relief of severe pain.

In a health context the Misuse of Drugs Regulations 2001 categorises controlled drugs into five numbered schedules.

- Schedule 1: No health purpose (e.g. lysergic acid).
- Schedule 2: Opiates (e.g. pethidine, diamorphine) and major stimulants (cocaine, amphetamines).
- Schedule 3: Barbiturates and minor stimulants (e.g. temazepam, one of the most widely abused prescription drugs in the UK, which is categorised for criminal purposes under Misuse of Drugs Regulation 2001 as a class C drug (class A if prepared for injection). It is an offence to possess or supply it without a prescription. Unlike the other benzodiazapines, it is therefore a schedule 3 drug for health purposes and subject to controlled drug prescribing and recording requirements).
- Schedule 4: Benzodiazapine tranquillisers, anabolic steroids.
- Schedule 5: Preparations with minimal risk of abuse.

Drugs from schedules 2 and 3 can only be dispensed on prescription. A valid prescription must be written indelibly, and must be dated and signed by the prescriber. The dose and name and address of the patient must be stated. For schedules 1 to 3 the dose of the drug must be in words and figures.

Special record-keeping requirements apply for controlled drugs. Drugs in schedules 1 and 2 of the 1985 regulations must have a record, kept in a bound register, each time the drug is obtained or supplied.

Midwives may possess and use specified controlled drugs under a midwives' supply order signed by a doctor or supervisor of midwives. The order must state the name and occupation of the midwife, why the drug is required and the total quantity to be obtained.

Currently, the Prescription Only Medicines (Human Use) Order 1997, schedule 5, allows a midwife to possess and administer diamorphine, morphine, pentazocine and pethidine hydrochloride when attending a woman in labour.

For schedule 2 controlled drugs the midwife must record supplies received and administered in a book solely used for that purpose. A midwife is not entitled to destroy surplus supplies of controlled drugs, but is able to surrender them to a medical officer identified in an agreed local policy.

A midwife might be in possession of controlled drugs as set out in the scenario below.

Scenario

A community midwife is preparing for a home confinement of a woman who required pethidine, a schedule 2 controlled drug, for pain relief during the birth of her previous child.

Under midwives' exemptions it is lawful for the midwife to possess and administer pethidine to a woman in labour without the need for a prescription.

The midwife obtains the drug for the delivery from the local pharmacist, using a supply order book signed by the supervisor of midwives. This is recorded in the midwife's controlled drug register and drug record book and the ampoules are securely stored in a locked container until required.

A healthy baby is delivered without the need for pethidine, which is returned to the supplying pharmacist. A record of the return is made in the midwife's controlled drug register and drug record book.

Professional requirements

Although the general legal requirements for the supply and administration of prescription-only medicines have exemptions for registered midwives, a midwife must have regard to her professional accountability and obligations when supplying or administering any medicines.

Midwives Rules and Standards

Through the *Midwives Rules and Standards* (NMC, 2004b) the NMC regulates a midwife's professional practice with regard to the supply and administration of medicines. While the rules acknowledge that midwives may be supplied with certain medicines listed in schedule 5 of the Prescription Only Medicines (Human Use) Order 1997, the regulatory body stresses that the actual drugs used by a midwife in practice must be agreed in a local policy in collaboration with a senior midwife, medical and pharmacy staff. Midwives are also required to limit the administration of medicines and dosages to those that they have been trained to use and administer.

Rule 7 requires that:

A practising midwife shall only supply and administer those medicines, including analgesics, in respect of which she [sic] has received the appropriate training as to use, dosage and methods of administration.

Professional requirements for medication management

The NMC sets out 26 standards for the management of medicines by midwives (NMC, 2008c). The standards for medicines management underpin the legal requirements that regulate the safety of medicines in the UK. It is essential that student midwives have a good working knowledge and are able to apply these standards in practice. Failing to meet the requirements of the NMC's *Standards for Medicines Management* could bring into question their fitness to practise, as illustrated by the following case study.

Scenario

A midwife stole 12 prescriptions belonging to a local medical centre and attempted to dishonestly obtain 30 temazepam tablets from a community pharmacy. She was convicted of both charges, given a probation order of 18 months and ordered to pay costs. She was also struck off the NMC Register.

Activity 13.4   *Research and group work*

Obtain a copy of the NMC's *Standards for Medicines Management* (2008c) from **www.nmc-uk.org** (navigate to publications, then standards and scroll to the relevant document).

* Discuss in a group how you would ensure that your use of medicines in practice reflects the requirements of the NMCs *Standards*.

As this activity will be based on your own discussion, there is no outline answer at the end of the chapter.

Midwives have a range of provisions under the law that allow them to supply and administer medicines, including some prescription-only and controlled drugs, in the course of their practice. Student midwives must become thoroughly familiar with medicines law and be able to apply the legislation to practice, in order to ensure the safety of the women and babies in their care.

C H A P T E R   S U M M A R Y

* Medicines make an important contribution to the therapeutic interventions used in healthcare.
* Medicines also have great potential to harm those who take them and are therefore regulated by the law.
* The purpose of using the law is to ensure that the right medicine is given to the right person at the right time in the right form and at the right dose.
* Initial statutory protection for all products is given by the Consumer Protection Act 1987.
* The principal statute regulating the use of medicines is the Medicines Act 1968.
* Before a drug can be marketed for sale or supply to the public, it must have a product licence or marketing authorisation.

- Drugs that have a manufacturing authorisation are categorised into three types for the purpose of supply to the general public: general sales list, pharmacy only and prescription only.
- Generally, prescription-only medicines can only be supplied against a valid prescription.
- Specific exemptions from restrictions on the supply or administration of prescription-only medicines under the Medicines Act 1968 are available to registered midwives.
- A patient group direction (PGD) is a written instruction for the supply or administration of a licensed medicine in an identified clinical situation where the patient may not be individually identified before presenting for treatment.
- A PGD is intended for local use and is a written instruction for medicines to be supplied for administering to a named patient.
- The regulations allow midwives who are prescribers to prescribe any licensed medicine, including issuing private prescriptions, for any medical condition that the midwife is competent to treat.
- Supplementary prescribing is a voluntary prescribing partnership between the independent prescriber and the supplementary prescriber to implement an agreed patient-specific clinical management plan.
- Controlled drugs are prescription-only medicines that are further regulated by the Misuse of Drugs Act 1971 because of their addictive properties.
- Currently, a midwife may possess and administer diamorphine, morphine, pentazocine and pethidine hydrochloride when attending a woman in labour.
- The NMC, through the *Midwives Rules and Standards* (2004b), regulates a midwife's professional practice with regard to the supply and administration of medicines.
- The NMC sets out some 26 standards for the management of medicines by midwives.
- Failing to meet the requirements of the NMC's *Standards for Medicines Management* (2008c) could bring into question a midwife's fitness to practise.

Knowledge review

Having completed the chapter, how would you now rate your knowledge of the following topics?

	Good	Adequate	Poor
1. The principal sources of law governing the safety of medicines.			
2. The three classifications of medicines used in the UK.			
3. The alternatives to prescription for the supply and administration of prescription-only medicines by midwives.			
4. The value to practice of midwives becoming non-medical prescribers.			

	Good	Adequate	Poor
5. The legal requirements for the possession and use of controlled drugs in midwifery practice.			

Where you're not confident in your knowledge of a topic, what will you do next?

Further reading

Jordan, S (ed.) (2009) *Pharmacology for Midwives: The evidence base for safe practice*, 2nd edn. London: Palgrave Macmillan.
This is a comprehensive pharmacology text that sets out the key medicines that midwives will use in practice.

Mason, JK and **Laurie, G** (2005) *Mason and McCall Smith's Law and Medical Ethics*, 7th edn. Oxford: Oxford University Press.
This is an advanced text that considers the ethical implications of healthcare law and contains a number of chapters on midwifery-related issues, such as reproduction law.

Useful websites

www.dh.gov.uk/en/Healthcare/Medicinespharmacyandindustry/Prescriptions/TheNon-MedicalPrescribingProgramme/index.htm The Department of Health's non-medical prescribing website, containing useful information about government policy on non-medical prescribing.
www.medicines.org.uk/emc The Electronic Medicines Compendium contains details, indications and common adverse reactions of every medicine licensed in the UK.
www.mhra.gov.uk The Medicines and Healthcare products Regulatory Agency approves new medicines and reports on adverse drug reactions. It gives up-to-date information on hazards, the development of new medicines and changes to medicines law.
www.nmc-uk.org Nursing and Midwifery Council, which provides a wide range of advice sheets and publications relating to medicines and midwifery. It is an essential source of information for all student midwives.
www.npc.co.uk The National Prescribing Centre supports high-quality, cost-effective prescribing and medicines management across the NHS to help improve patient care and service delivery.

Chapter 14

Health and safety

NMC Standards for Pre-registration Midwifery Education

This chapter will address the following competency:

Domain: Professional and ethical practice

- Support the creation and maintenance of environments that promote the health, safety and wellbeing of women, babies and others. This will include:
  - Promoting health, safety and security in the environment in which the midwife is working, whether it be at a woman's home, in the community, a clinic, or in a hospital.

Chapter aims

After reading this chapter, you will be able to:

- state why health and safety matters should concern registered midwives;
- outline the general duties owed by employers and employees under the Health and Safety at Work etc. Act 1974;
- describe the regulations governing specific health and safety requirements in the NHS;
- explain the process of health and safety management;
- discuss the requirements for the safe handling of loads;
- define the term 'reasonably practicable' in relation to manual handling;
- discuss the lawfulness of no-lift policy in relation to practice.

Introduction

There is no argument that midwives' health and safety, and that of women in their care, should be given serious consideration at all times. Therefore, right at the start of students' midwifery preparation programmes, their universities and clinical placements will be concerned for their safety and the safety of those they care for. In this chapter, we will explore the duties owed by healthcare employers and their staff under health and safety legislation. The process of safety management and, in particular, the requirements for the safe handling of loads will be considered. The chapter ends with a discussion of the human rights impact of health and safety laws.

As the UK's largest employer, the NHS has over 1.7 million employees who directly or indirectly provide care and treatment for nearly 11 million people a year. About 25,500 midwives are employed by the NHS to provide antenatal care, care during labour and postnatal care (National Statistics, 2008), Therefore, ensuring the health and safety of all employees is essential to the efficient delivery of healthcare for all.

Activity 14.1   *Reflection*

- In a group list the potential risks to your health and safety that you have encountered during clinical practice.
- When you have completed this, make another list of the potential hazards faced by mothers and babies receiving healthcare.

Please do not move on to the next part until you are ready for the answer.

A report commissioned by the Department of Health in 2008 found that nearly half of all staff absence in the NHS is accounted for by musculoskeletal disorders and more than a quarter by stress, depression and anxiety, costing the NHS 1.7 billion pounds (DH, 2009). The report has recommended a new health and safety strategy for NHS staff, with a potential saving of £555 million for the taxpayer.

According to the Health and Safety Executive (HSE, 2010), absences in the NHS are caused by four main types of accidents.

- **Musculoskeletal disorders** (along with stress) are the biggest cause of sick leave in the NHS, accounting for some 40 per cent of all sick leave. For example, an average of seven midwives suffered work-related musculoskeletal disorder annually in 2006–08.
- **Stress** is a major cause of work-related ill health and sick leave among healthcare employees. Work-related stress accounts for over a third of all new incidences of ill health and each case leads to an average of 30.2 working days lost. A total of 13.8 million working days were lost to work-related stress, depression and anxiety in 2006–07.
- **Slips and trips** were responsible for 54 per cent of major injuries in healthcare in 2007–08.
- **Violence** is experienced by NHS staff and other healthcare workers four times more commonly than by other workers. Employers must assess the risk of verbal and physical violence to their employees and take appropriate steps to deal with it.

CASE STUDY: Woman bit midwife

A woman was jailed for 20 weeks for deliberately biting a midwife helping to deliver her baby. She was in the final stages of labour when she sank her teeth into the forearm of the experienced midwife. Despite needing immediate first aid, the midwife went back on to the ward to help the young woman give birth. But she later had to endure six months of HIV and hepatitis tests because the mother was a high-risk patient (*Daily Mail*, 2010).

Those receiving healthcare are also placed at risk of injury if appropriate health and safety measures are not taken. Data from the National Patient Safety Agency (NPSA, 2009) have shown that there were more than 700,000 'patient safety incidents' in the NHS in 2006–07. The NHS Litigation Authority (2009) estimates that some £500 million is paid annually by the health service in compensation claims and fines for breaching health and safety laws. The cost in human terms can also be high when lives are put at risk and fatalities occur. The case below illustrates how a breach in health and safety can affect those receiving healthcare and this can include pregnant women.

CASE STUDY: Patient falls from window

An NHS Trust was fined after admitting breaching health and safety legislation when a vulnerable and partially sighted patient fell from a first-floor window at a hospital. Restricters that should have been in place to prevent the window opening wide enough for a person to jump out had not been fitted. The Trust in question had failed in its duty to ensure the health and safety of the patient, who was left severely injured after a fall that should never have happened (HSE, 2009).

Health and safety law

As an employer, the NHS has a legal duty to comply with the requirements relating to the health and safety of its employees and those using the service, in order to prevent injuries and avoidable loss of life.

The Health and Safety at Work etc. Act 1974 is the basis of health and safety law in the UK. It sets out general duties that:

- employers have towards employees and members of the public using their service;
- employees have to themselves and to each other.

Breaching or failing to comply with these duties are criminal offences.

The employer's general duty is set out in section 2 of the Health and Safety at Work etc. Act 1974:

Duty to ensure so far as is reasonably practicable, the health, safety and welfare at work of employees and any others who may be affected by the undertaking.

The legal standard imposed by the 1974 Act is *reasonably practicable* or *so far as is reasonably practicable*. The standard implies a weighing up of the risk against the cost, in terms of time, money or trouble, of preventing or controlling the risk.

In the case of new and expectant mothers, where risks are identified, the mother is entitled to a change in working conditions or an offer of suitable alternative work. Where this is not possible, she can be suspended from work on full pay for as long as is necessary.

The duty of employees at work is set out in section 7 of the Health and Safety at Work etc. Act 1974, which states that it shall be the duty of every employee while at work:

- to take reasonable care of their own health and safety and of any other person who may be affected by their acts or omissions;

- to cooperate with their employer so far as is necessary to enable that employer to meet their requirements with regard to any statutory provisions.

Duty to report incidents

As well as a duty under the Health and Safety at Work etc. Act 1974, registered midwives are also under a professional duty to act to identify and minimise the risk to colleagues and those under their care (NMC, 2004a).

A midwife who raises an issue of health and safety with an employer either directly or through a union is entitled to protection from dismissal and victimisation under the Public Interest Disclosure Act 1998. Under the Act, each NHS employer has a duty to establish a procedure for employees to raise concerns where:

- a criminal offence has been, is being or is likely to be committed; or
- the health or safety of an individual has been, is being or is likely to be endangered.

Health and safety regulations

The Health and Safety at Work etc. Act 1974 is supplemented by a wide range of secondary legislation in the form of regulations and orders (see Table 14.1). These focus on specific areas of workplace health and safety, such as manual handling. Most of this secondary legislation begins in the form of an EU directive, which must be implemented in the law of individual member states. The directives aim to harmonise workplace health and safety throughout the countries of the EU.

It is essential that employers and staff work together to ensure effective implementation of health and safety measures. This joint approach helps to promote and raise awareness of health and safety among employers and staff, thereby creating a positive safety culture.

Involving staff in workplace health and safety is a legal requirement under the provisions of the Safety Representatives and Safety Committee Regulations 1977 and the Health and Safety (Consultation with Employees) Regulations 1996. These require staff representatives to:

- consult with, and be consulted by, employers regarding:
  - the introduction of measures that may affect health and safety;
  - arrangements for appointing competent persons to assess risks and provision of health and safety information and training;
  - investigation of hazards, accidents and complaints etc.;
- make representation to the employer on health and safety matters;
- perform workplace inspections;
- be given time off to perform their duties and undertake health and safety training.

Table 14.1: Regulations relating to health and safety in the NHS

Regulations	Scope
Management of Health and Safety at Work Regulations 1999	Set out how employers are required to assess risk in all work activities, implement control measures if required, provide information and training, and appoint competent persons.
Manual Handling Operations Regulations 1992	Cover the moving and handling of objects either by hand or by bodily force.
Control of Substances Hazardous to Health Regulations 2002	Relate to the assessment of hazardous substances and biological agents and the implementation of appropriate precautions.
Reporting of Injuries, Diseases and Dangerous Occurrences Regulations 1995	Require employers to notify certain types of injury, disease and dangerous occurrences to the Health and Safety Executive.
Personal Protective Equipment at Work Regulations 1992	Cover the provision of suitable and sufficient protective clothing and equipment, such as uniforms and gloves.
Workplace (Health, Safety and Welfare) Regulations 1992	Cover issues such as ventilation, temperature, flooring and workstations.
The Health and Safety (Display Screen Equipment) Regulations 1992	Set out requirements for the use of visual display units, workstations, seating, etc.
Provision and Use of Work Equipment Regulations 1998	Cover the safe use and maintenance of equipment, such as hoists, at work.
Health and Safety (First Aid) Regulations 1981	Concern first aid requirements, such as the contents of first aid boxes and the number of trained first aid personnel.
The Health and Safety (Safety Signs and Signals) Regulations 1996	Specify the minimum requirements for safety signs at work.
The Fire Precautions (Workplaces) Regulations 1997	Require employers to assess the risk of fire in the workplace.
Hazardous Waste (England and Wales) Regulations 2005	Specify the requirements for the classification, segregation and disposal of waste, including infectious and hazardous waste.

Managing health and safety

The HSE (2006) requires workplace health and safety to be managed methodically to ensure that risks are minimised. This includes establishing a health and safety policy to provide information on the management of work-related risks. The policy will complement the Trust's policies that relate to specific requirements, such as manual handling and the control of substances hazardous to health.

It also includes demonstrating that health and safety management is organised and functioning by reference to the four Cs.

- **Cooperation**:
  - good safety performance depends on everyone cooperating and safety is everybody's business;
  - there is a legal requirement to consult with staff representatives on health and safety matters.
- **Communication**:
  - consultation with staff safety representatives;
  - performing workplace inspections at regular intervals with written reports available for staff to view;
  - setting up a workplace Safety Committee.
- **Control**:
  - there is a legal requirement to exercise control of health and safety to ensure compliance. If there is failure to comply with an identified safety rule, such as not disposing of clinical waste appropriately, and action is not taken to rectify the situation, both the employer and staff member break the law.
- **Competence**:
  - employees must have the knowledge and skills needed to work without risk to themselves or to others who come into contact with their work;
  - managers must ensure that individuals for whom they are responsible have the appropriate skills and knowledge to work without risk to themselves or to others;
  - competence is a legal requirement imposed on employers through health and safety regulations; training in health and safety measures is a mandatory component of a health service contract.

Activity 14.3 — Group work

- In a group discuss which elements of your midwifery education programme might be considered to be health and safety training, for example manual handling training. Make a list of the topics covered.
- Now compare that list with the list of hazards you identified in Activity 14.1 at the start of this chapter. Does the training reflect the hazards you are likely to encounter in the course of your practice?

Please do not move on to the next part until you are ready for the answer.

Assessment and monitoring risks

The risks associated with performing workplace tasks must be assessed, along with identification of any workplace precautions and risk control systems that may be required and their successful implementation. Inspections and risk assessments must be monitored.

Review and audit

Performance must be reviewed against an audit of documentation, such as workplace inspections, risk assessments and accident and incident reports, and attendance on health and safety training courses.

Health and safety inspectors

Health and safety inspectors are employed by the HSE to ensure that health and safety duties are implemented. The inspectors have the power to inspect premises, such as a hospital, and take enforcement action, such as improvement or prohibition notices relating to health and safety issues. They can order that the premises or equipment are made safe and they can order that a particular activity is stopped until the hazards or dangers are removed. The inspectors have the power to prosecute for failure to comply with a health and safety notice or for breach of health and safety duties.

CASE STUDY: Latex allergy

In *Dugmore v Swansea NHS Trust* [2002], a health professional was awarded £345,000 from her employing Trust for injuries caused by hazardous substances. In 1997, she was forced to abandon her career due to an allergy to latex after experiencing asthma, skin problems and anaphylactic attacks after exposure to latex.

The Trust was liable because, although it had taken the step of providing the health professional with latex-free products, other staff on the ward continued to use them and this was enough to trigger an allergic reaction.

Workplace risk assessments

A risk assessment is the identification of hazards present in the workplace and an estimate of the risk associated with performing a task. A hazard is something that has the potential to cause harm and a risk is the likelihood of that hazard causing an accident or incident.

Workplace should be interpreted in its widest sense. For example, midwives may attend childbearing women whatever the setting, and a woman's home could therefore be classed as a work setting for midwives.

CASE STUDY: Community midwife attacked

A midwife on call to attend a newborn baby was viciously attacked when leaving the family home and returning to her car (*Peterborough Today*, 2008). The attacker pounced on her, knocked her to the floor in the stairwell, rendering her semi-conscious, and stole her medical bag and ID card. Following the incident, the Trust issued attack alarms to all community midwives who look after mothers and babies in their own homes.

Commenting on the incident, the Royal College of Midwives expected the Trust to carry out a risk assessment to protect midwives and not breach health and safety rules.

It is important for employers to carry out a risk assessment in the workplace in order to protect their employees. Failure to do so may result in employees being exposed to unnecessary hazards, with serious human cost and employers being penalised financially. The following case illustrates the cost to healthcare workers, including midwives, and monetary cost where health and safety rules are breached.

Scenario

An experienced midwife was working in the delivery suite in the local hospital. This work involved heavy manual handling of patients. She had a long history of back complaints and a small disc prolapse in her lower spine. Her employer did not send her to their occupational health department to assess her fitness for the work in the delivery suite, despite being told of her back problems. The manual handling work in the delivery suite aggravated the lower-back problem and increased the disc prolapse, such that she had to have surgery within one year and was retired on grounds of ill health.

The court found that the hospital had failed to carry out a risk assessment and was therefore in breach of its statutory duties and also negligent.

There is a legal duty to perform risk assessments under the provisions of the Management of Health and Safety at Work Regulations 1999.

Once a hazard has been identified, the likelihood of the risk occurring and the severity of the harm must be considered. The law requires that risks should be reduced *so far as is reasonably practicable*. That means that the degree of risk should be balanced against the time, trouble, cost and physical difficulty of taking measures to avoid it.

On identifying a risk, steps must be taken to minimise it by:

- elimination of the hazard at source; if this is not possible, the hazard must be reduced;
- taking action, if the hazard can only be reduced, to control the risk by introducing workplace precautions such as alarms, training information;
- putting in place, once workplace precautions have been introduced, a system to monitor compliance.

For example, the Control of Substances Hazardous to Health Regulations 2002 seek to control exposure to hazardous substances that arise out of work under an employer's control. Under Regulation 7(1), exposure of employees to substances hazardous to health must either be prevented or, where this is not reasonably practicable, adequately controlled. Therefore, employers must, where reasonably practicable, eliminate completely the use or production of substances hazardous to health in the workplace by changing the method of work, modifying the process or substituting with a non-hazardous substance.

Where prevention of exposure to substances hazardous to health is not reasonably practicable, employers must adequately control exposure.

Reporting accidents and incidents

Reporting accidents and incidents at work is an essential component of monitoring the effectiveness of health and safety measures and preventing recurrence of an incident. In addition to local NHS Trust accident-reporting procedures, there is a legal requirement to report certain categories of accidents that occur within the workplace to the HSE under the Reporting of Injuries, Diseases and Dangerous Occurrences Regulations 1995 (RIDDOR).

Accidents at work are only reportable if they arise out of, or in connection with, work. The different categories of accidents are as follows.

- **Death or major injuries**: accidents that are reportable when a member of staff (while working) or someone receiving healthcare is killed or suffers a major injury. This includes injuries sustained as a result of physical violence. It also includes injuries sustained when working in a community setting.
- **Injuries lasting over three days**: accidents (including acts of physical violence) that result in the injured person being away from work or unable to perform their normal duties for more than three days (including non-working days).
- **Diseases**: where a doctor notifies a Trust in writing that an employee is suffering from a disease specified in regulations and linked with a workplace activity, this incident must be reported. Reportable diseases include:
  - occupational dermatitis;
  - occupational asthma or respiratory sensitisation as a result of exposure to chemical substances;
  - infections such as hepatitis, tuberculosis, legionella and tetanus;
  - infection reliably attributable to working with biological agents – exposure to blood or body fluids or any potentially infective material.

Dangerous occurrences

Dangerous occurrences or near misses must also be reported and are events that may not result in a reportable injury, but have the potential to do significant harm. In the health service reportable occurrences would include:

- collapse, overturning or failure of load-bearing parts of lifts and lifting equipment, such as a hoist;
- explosion, collapse or bursting of any closed vessel or associated pipe work, such as an autoclave;
- electrical short circuit or overload causing fire or explosion;
- explosion or fire causing suspension of normal work for over 24 hours;
- accidental release of any substance that may damage health, including blood spillage.

Manual handling

The risk of injury

Musculoskeletal injury, particularly back injury, is one of the most common causes of incapacity among healthcare professionals. Midwives are at risk due to the range of manual handling activities undertaken during the course of their practice. Of the 12,000 reported serious injuries to healthcare staff, in excess of 50 per cent relate to moving and handling (HSE, 2004). In the NHS, 40 per cent of sickness absence relates to manual handling accidents, costing £400 million every year (DH, 2002).

Reducing the risk of injury

The Management of Health and Safety at Work Regulations 1999 require employers to make an assessment of the risks to the health and safety of their employees and others they have contact with in work. The regulations further require that protective and preventative measures be put in place to avoid such risks.

The Manual Handling Operations Regulations 1992 deal specifically with the manual handling of loads. Regulation 2(1) defines manual handling as *any transporting or supporting of a load (including the lifting, putting down, pushing, pulling, carrying or moving thereof) by hand or by bodily force*. A load is defined as including *any person and any animal*. Therefore, the scope of the regulations includes the lifting and moving of those being cared for by midwifery staff.

Regulation 4 of the 1992 regulations places a duty on employers to avoid hazardous manual handling operations as far as is reasonably practicable. Where this cannot be avoided, the regulation requires an assessment of the operation and steps to be taken to reduce the risk of injury to the lowest level reasonably practicable. Particular consideration should be given to the provision of mechanical assistance, such as hoists, but where this is not reasonably practicable employers should explore improvements to the task, the load and the working environment.

Both the general duty to protect the health and safety of employees and the specific duty to reduce risks to health due to the manual handling of loads apply to the health service.

CASE STUDY: Failing to comply with manual handling regulations

In *Knott v Newham Health Care Trust* [2002], a health professional brought a claim against her Trust for damages for a back injury, arguing that the injury resulted from the manual handling of people without appropriate training, equipment and assistance. She suffered lower back pain, urinary incontinence and sensory disturbances in the legs and was unable to sit for more than 15 minutes. The Trust submitted that she had exaggerated her symptoms and that the damage was constitutional in nature.

The court found that the lifting equipment provided by the Trust was inadequate to protect staff from injury and that the Trust had failed to make a proper assessment of the risk of injury. The absence of mechanical lifting aids meant that staff resorted to manual methods, which carried an inherent and well-publicised risk of injury. The court awarded £45,000 in damages.

No-lift policies

Activity 14.4   *Critical thinking*

Before reading this section, read the manual handling policy of the NHS Trust you attend for clinical practice. Note the requirements of the policy. Does it allow any form of lifting or moving of patients by manual means?

Please do not move on to the next part until you are ready for the answer.

As current national guidelines now advocate a 'no-lift policy' where patient handling is concerned, a vast number of Trusts have adopted this policy in relation to manual handling. No-lift policy is seen as a means of reducing injury when handling patients and the advice from many professional bodies, including the RCM, is that hazardous manual handling should be eliminated in all but exceptional or life-threatening situations. NHS Trusts and trade unions representing staff in the health service see the use of a no-lift policy as the key tool in reducing manual handling injuries. Instead of lifting manually, these policies require that the great majority of lifting is achieved by mechanical means.

Reasonably practicable

Despite the liability NHS Trusts face under statutory health and safety provisions, the duty is not absolute. The Health and Safety at Work etc. Act 1974 and its regulations only require the duties to be carried out as far as is reasonably practicable.

The meaning of this phrase was considered by the Court of Appeal in *Edwards v National Coal Board* [1949]. Lord Justice Asquith held that reasonably practicable did not mean physically possible. NHS Trusts are not required to spend all their funds on ensuring the safety of staff. Rather, there is a narrower requirement to balance the likelihood of the risk occurring against the cost in terms of money, time and trouble in averting the risk. In manual handling terms this has generally been considered to be balancing the risk of injury to staff against the cost and availability of suitable equipment. The rights and preferences of patients were considered secondary to the primary duty of protecting the health and safety of staff. Under no-lift policies, patients would not be moved or lifted if manual handling was assessed as hazardous and suitable equipment was not available.

Activity 14.5   *Research and group work*

To help you to apply the legal concepts introduced in the next section of this chapter, download and read *R (on the application of A & Others) v East Sussex County Council & Another* [2003] EWHC 167 from **www.bailii.org/ew/cases/EWHC/Admin/2003/167.html**.

- In a group discuss the facts of the case and whether you agree with the outcome of the case.

Please do not move on to the next part until you are ready for the answer.

When the Human Rights Act 1998 was introduced, the High Court revisited the interpretation of reasonably practicable and now requires the rights of patients to be considered when assessing moving and handling needs.

Concept summary: Assessing reasonable practicability

R (on the application of A & Others) v East Sussex County Council & Another [2003] EWHC 167 (Admin)

In assessing what is reasonably practicable the approach is as follows:

a) the possible methods of avoiding or minimising the risk must be considered (in practice the only alternative to manual lifting in a case such as this is likely to be a hoist);

   b) the context – the frequency and duration of the manoeuvres – must be considered: the assessment must be based on the pattern of lifting over a period (typically a day), not on an individual lift basis – a particular lift might be done manually if done only once a day but not if required frequently during the day;

   c) the risks to the employee in question associated with each of the possible methods must be assessed: there must be an analysis of:

      i)   the likelihood of any injury to the employee; and

      ii) the severity of any injury to the employee;

   d) the impact upon the person, physical, emotional, psychological or social, of each of the possible methods of avoiding manual lifting must be examined: there must be an analysis of:

      i)   the physical and mental personality and characteristics of the person and their personality – this necessarily includes the nature and degree of disablement;

      ii) the wishes and feelings of the person: any evinced negative reaction in the nature of dislike, reluctance, fear, refusal or other manifestation of negative attitude is relevant, though not of course determinative;

      iii) the effect upon the person's dignity and rights, including in particular their rights (protected by article 8) to physical and psychological integrity, to respect for their privacy, to develop their personality and to go out into the community and meet others and their right (protected by article 3) to be free from inhuman or degrading treatment.

These considerations will necessarily involve assessing the impact upon the person of carrying out a manoeuvre other than a manual lift in terms of considerations of personal dignity or the amount of respect afforded to their persons, their quality of life generally – their ability to spend their time in activities other than merely performing bodily functions – and, importantly, matters such as their access to the community.

The assessment must be focused on the particular circumstances of the individual case. Just as context is everything, so the individual assessment is all. Thus, for example:

   a) the assessment must take into account the particular person's personal physical and mental characteristics, be 'user focused' and 'user led' and should be part of the wider care-planning process for that particular individual;

   b) there must be an assessment of the particular person's autonomy interests;

   c) the assessment must be based on the particular workers involved (not workers in the abstract);

   d) the assessment must be based on the pattern of lifting in the particular case.

Duty to the women in a midwife's care

At common law patients are owed a duty of care that requires that health professionals meet their needs in accordance with a standard accepted by a responsible body of professional opinion and that stands up to logical analysis (*Bolitho v City & Hackney HA* [1998]). In midwifery practice, meeting this duty may require the manual handling of pregnant women even where there is a risk of injury.

The common law duty of care requires that a person whose job includes lifting people accepts a greater risk than those whose handling duty is restricted to inanimate objects. Therefore, in midwifery practice the care of women gives rise to an inherent need for some manual handling to take place.

Human rights issues

A duty to those being cared for by midwives may also arise if rights under the Human Rights Act 1998 are engaged. Article 2 of the European Convention on Human Rights places a positive obligation on states to protect life. Therefore, there would be a duty to manually lift a person away from danger if this were the only method of removal available. Where no-lift policies totally prohibit any manual handling, it will be a breach of article 2 of the Convention and would be unlawful.

Article 3 of the Convention prohibits, without exception, torture, inhuman or degrading treatment. What constitutes inhuman or degrading treatment is a matter of fact and degree in each case. It can occur through thoughtless and uncaring actions. To confine to her bed a pregnant woman who is unable to move unaided, without the opportunity to use the bathroom for her toilet and washing needs, could be a breach of article 3. No-lift policies that forbid manual handling in such conditions would be unlawful.

Human rights obligations may also arise in handling situations under article 8 of the Convention. Unlike the right to life and the right to freedom from inhuman or degrading treatment, rights under article 8 are not absolute, but qualified. This means that the countervailing rights of midwives and carers must also be considered.

Everyone is owed a duty of respect for their dignity and, in circumstances where this may be lost, that duty requires action to be taken. A duty of respect for dignity would require, by manual means if necessary, action to restore the individual's dignity. That is not to say that handling a person by mechanical means is inherently undignified. Nor is the respect for dignity absolute. There are circumstances when caring for or treating a person requires undignified means to achieve a dignified end. This is recognised by the European Court of Human Rights, which held that a measure that is convincingly shown to be a therapeutic necessity cannot be a breach of articles 3 or 8 of the Convention (*Herczegfalvy v Austria* (1993)).

A handling situation that gave rise to the pregnant woman's right to respect for physiological and psychological integrity would also require respect for the midwife's physiological and psychological integrity. It is clear, therefore, that in circumstances where article 8 rights are engaged a balance needs to be struck between the rights of the pregnant woman and the rights of the midwife.

Where someone has a longer-term disability that requires lifting to ensure social interaction and contact with the community, the Court further held that it would be unlawful to deny the person access on the grounds that mechanical lifting was not available. The Court cited examples such as failing to take a person out because a power cut meant a hoist could not be used, or restricting time for activities because either a hoist was not available or continence management away from the place of residence required manual handling (*R (on the application of A & Others) v East Sussex County Council & Another* [2003]).

CHAPTER SUMMARY

- The NHS employs some 1.7 million people and treats over 11 million people a year. This includes 24,600 midwives providing antenatal care, care during labour and postnatal care. Therefore, ensuring the health and safety of all employees is essential to the efficient delivery of healthcare for all.
- It is essential to safeguard the health and safety of these employees in order that efficient healthcare can be delivered.
- The HSE estimates that absence in the NHS costs some £1 billion annually.
- Women and their babies are also placed at risk of injury if appropriate safety measures are not taken.
- The basis of health and safety law in the UK is the Health and Safety at Work etc. Act 1974.
- An employer has a duty to ensure, so far as is reasonably practicable, the health, safety and welfare at work of employees and any others who may be affected by the undertaking.
- Employees at work have a duty to take reasonable care of their own health and safety and that of any other person who may be affected by their acts or omissions.
- The Health and Safety at Work etc. Act 1974 is supplemented by a wide range of secondary legislation in the form of regulations that focus on specific areas of workplace health and safety.
- Employers and staff must work together to ensure effective implementation of health and safety measures.
- The HSE requires workplace health and safety to be managed methodically to ensure that risks are minimised.
- There is a legal duty to perform risk assessments under the provisions of the Management of Health and Safety at Work Regulations 1999.
- The Control of Substances Hazardous to Health Regulations 2002 control exposure to hazardous substances that arise out of work.
- It is a legal requirement to report certain accidents that occur in the workplace to the HSE under the Reporting of Injuries, Diseases and Dangerous Occurrences Regulations 1995 (RIDDOR).
- Musculoskeletal injury, particularly back injury, is one of the most common causes of incapacity among nurses and midwives.
- The Manual Handling Operations Regulations 1992 deal specifically with the manual handling of loads.
- There will be circumstances where the risk to the woman or her baby, if not lifted, will override the midwife's ordinary health and safety concerns, even where manual handling would be considered hazardous.
- In the case of hazardous handling situations, manual handling will be the exception rather than the rule.

Knowledge review

Having completed the chapter, how would you now rate your knowledge of the following topics?

	Good	Adequate	Poor
1. The relationship between midwifery and health and safety law.			
2. The general duties owed by employers and employees under the Health and Safety at Work etc. Act 1974.			
3. The regulations governing specific health and safety requirements in the NHS.			
4. The process of health and safety management.			
5. The requirements for the safe handling of loads.			
6 The term 'reasonably practicable' in relation to manual handling.			

Where you're not confident in your knowledge of a topic, what will you do next?

Further reading

For a fuller discussion of the health and safety risks to staff we recommend:

National Audit Office (2003) *A Safer Place to Work: Improving the management of health and safety risks to staff in NHS Trusts* (House of Commons Papers). London: NAO.

Useful websites

www.hse.gov.uk   The Health and Safety Executive's role is to prevent death, injury and ill health to those at work and those affected by work activities, including the NHS. It provides a wide range of information about health and safety and even takes the time each month to counter the many myths that spread about health and safety law.

www.npsa.nhs.uk   The National Patient Safety Agency leads and contributes to improving safe patient care by informing, supporting and influencing the health sector.

References

Attewill, F (2007) Jehovah's Witness mother dies after refusing blood transfusion. *The Guardian*, 5 May.

Audit Commission (1999) *Setting the Record Straight*. London: Audit Commission.

Bainham, A (1990) *Children: The new law*. London: Family Law.

Ballinger, L (2010) Illegal immigrant gets life for killing 6 weeks old daughter. *Daily Mail*, 20 February, p6.

Beauchamp, T and Childress, J (1989) *Principles of Biomedical Ethics*. Oxford: Oxford University Press.

Bellis, G (2005) Carer jailed for sex assault on mental patient. *Liverpool Daily Post*, 5 August, p2.

Bewley, S, Friend, JR and Mezey, GC (1997) *Violence Against Women*. London: RCOG Press.

Bourke, F (2005) Nurse accused of raping OAP is struck off. *Sunday Mercury*, 16 July, p21.

Brady, E (2008) £8 million payout for Dudley boy disabled by medical failure. *Birmingham Post*, 1 July, p1.

Britten, N (2007) Jury finds mother guilty of aborting foetus at 30 weeks. *The Daily Telegraph*, 27 May, p8.

Butler-Sloss, E (2003) *Are We Failing the Family? Human rights, children and the meaning of family in the 21st century*. London: Department for Constitutional Affairs.

Care Quality Commission (CQC) (2009) *Safeguarding Children: A review of arrangements in the NHS for safeguarding children*. London: CQC.

Carruthers, I and Ormondroyd, J (2009) *Achieving Age Equality in Health and Social Care*. London: Central Office of Information.

Cox, AR and Ferner, RE (2009) Prescribing errors in diabetes. *British Journal of Diabetes Vascular Disease*, 9: 84–8.

Craft, N (1996) BMA issues new guidance on surrogacy. *British Medical Journal*, 312: 397–8.

Crow, L (2003) Invisible and centre stage: a disabled woman's perspective on maternity services. *RCM Midwives*, 6(4): 158–61.

Crown Prosecution Service (CPS) (2004) *The Code for Crown Prosecutors*. London: CPS.

Daily Mail (2010) Young mother jailed for biting midwife during childbirth, 6 February, p7.

De Bruxelles, S (2010) Hospital admits guilt over labour death of Mayra Cabrera. *The Times*, 5 March, p4.

Department for Constitutional Affairs (2007) *Mental Capacity Act 2005 Code of Practice*. London: The Stationery Office.

Department of Health (DH) (1997a) *Children Act 1989: Guidance and regulations*. London: HMSO.

Department of Health (DH) (1997b) *On the State of the Public Health: The annual report of the chief medical officer.* London: Department of Health.

Department of Health (DH) (1999) *Working Together to Safeguard Children.* London: The Stationery Office.

Department of Health (DH) (2000) *Domestic Violence: A resource manual for health care professionals.* London: Department of Health.

Department of Health (DH) (2002) *No Secrets: Guidance on developing and implementing multi-agency policies and procedures to protect vulnerable adults from abuse.* London: The Stationery Office.

Department of Health (DH) (2003a) *Confidentiality: NHS code of practice.* London: Department of Health.

Department of Health (DH) (2003b) *Every Child Matters* (Cmnd 5860). London: The Stationery Office.

Department of Health (DH) (2003c) *The Victoria Climbié Inquiry* (Lord Laming, Cmnd 5730). London: The Stationery Office

Department of Health (DH) (2004) *Independent Investigation into How the NHS Handled Allegations about the Conduct of Clifford Ayling* (The Honourable Mrs Justice Pauffley, Cmnd 6298). London: Department of Health.

Department of Health (DH) (2009) *NHS Health & Wellbeing Final Report.* London: Department of Health.

Department of Health and Social Security (DHSS) (1984) *Report of the Committee of Inquiry into Human Fertilisation and Embryology* (Dame Mary Warnock, Cmnd 9314). London: HMSO.

Department of Health/Department for Children, Schools and Families (DH/DCSF) (2009) *Getting Maternity Services Right for Pregnant Teenagers and Young Fathers*, 2nd edn. London: DCSF.

Department of Health/Office of National Statistics (DH/ONS) (2009) *Abortion Statistics, England and Wales: 2008.* London: Department of Health.

Dimond, B (2006) What is the law if a patient refuses treatment based on the nurse's race? *British Journal of Nursing*, 15(19): 1077–8.

Douglas, G (1993) *Law, Fertility and Reproduction.* London: Sweet and Maxwell.

Dyer, O (2002) GMC reprimands consultant for terminating pregnancy without consent. *British Medical Journal*, 324: 1354.

Edwards, S (2009) *Nursing Ethics: A principle-based approach*, 2nd edn. Basingstoke: Palgrave.

Emlyn, S (ed.) (1971) *Hale's History of the Pleas of the Crown.* London: Professional Books.

Equality and Human Rights Commission (EHRC) (2007) *Interim Business Plan 2007–08.* London: EHRC.

European Commission (2007) *Developing a Community Framework for Safe, High Quality and Efficient Health Services.* Brussels: European Commission.

Evening Gazette (2006) Struck off, 31 January, p5.

Foreign and Commonwealth Office (FCO) (2007) *Dealing with Cases of Forced Marriage. Practice guidance for health professionals.* London: The Stationery Office.

Foreign and Commonwealth Office (FCO) (2008) *The Right to Choose: Multiagency statutory guidance for dealing with forced marriages.* London: The Stationery Office.

FORWARD (2007) *A Statistical Study to Estimate the Prevalence of Female Genital Mutilation in England and Wales.* London: FORWARD.

Gillon, R (1994) Medical ethics: four principles plus attention to scope. *British Medical Journal*, 309: 184.

Grear, A (2004) The curate, a cleft palate and ideological closure in the Abortion Act 1967 – time to reconsider the relationship between doctors and the abortion decision. *Web Journal of Current Legal Issues*, 4. Available online at http://webjcli.ncl.ac.uk/2004/issue4/grear4.html (accessed 1 June 2010).

Green, C (2008) Fears for British doctor held captive by relatives. *The Independent*, 9 December.

Hampshire and Isle of Wight Counter Fraud Team (2007) Student midwife starts jail sentence. *Fraud Matters*, June, p1.

Hansard (1990) House of Lords, vol. 522, col. 1039.

Health and Safety Executive (HSE) (2004) *Health and Safety Statistics Highlights*. London: HSE.

Health and Safety Executive (HSE) (2006) *Five Steps to Risk Assessment*. London: HSE.

Health and Safety Executive (HSE) (2009) Primary Care Trust fined £10,000 after patient falls 4 metres from window. Press Release HSE/E/31. London: HSE.

Health and Safety Executive (HSE) (2010) *Health and Safety in Health and Social Care Services*. London: HSE.

HM Government (2006) *Working Together to Safeguard Children*. London: The Stationery Office.

Home Office (1990) *Domestic Violence* (Circular 60/90). London: Home Office.

Home Office (2002) *Protecting the Public: Strengthening protection against sex offenders and reforming the law on sexual offences* (Cmnd 5668). London: The Stationery Office.

Home Office (2004) *Tackling Domestic Violence: The role of health professionals*. London: The Stationery Office.

Home Office (2005) *Crime in England & Wales 2004/05*. London: The Stationery Office.

Home Office (2009) *Crime in England & Wales 2008/09*. London: The Stationery Office.

Human Fertilisation and Embryology Authority (HFEA) (2003) HFEA issues guidance on egg giving (Press release). Available online at www.hfea.gov.uk/797.html (accessed 1 June 2010).

John, P (2005) Bringing joy and heartache to women. *Birmingham Evening Mail*, 30 September, p2.

Jordan, S (ed.) (2009) *Pharmacology for Midwives: The evidence base for safe practice*, 2nd edn. London: Palgrave Macmillan.

Kennedy, I and Grubb, A (1998) *Principles of Medical Law*. Oxford: Oxford University Press.

Knowles, K (2009) Midwife who stood by as a baby's head turned blue. *Bedfordshire*, 15 March, p2.

Lancashire Telegraph (2009) Bungling midwife tells hearing of her regret, 26 May, p2.

Law Commission (1992) *Domestic Violence and Occupation of the Family Home* (Report No. 207). London: HMSO.

Law Commission (1993) *Mentally Incapacitated and Other Vulnerable Adults: Public law protection* (Consultation Paper 130). London: The Stationery Office.

Lazenbatt, A (2010) Safeguarding children and public health: midwives' responsibilities. *Perspectives in Public Health*, 130(3): 118–26.

Lewis, F and Batey, M (1982) Clarifying autonomy and accountability in nursing services. *Journal of Nursing Administration*, 12(9): 13–18.

Macpherson, Sir William (1999) *Stephen Lawrence Inquiry*. London: The Stationery Office.

Manchester Evening News (2003) Midwife in racist row escapes jail, 30 July.

Manchester Evening News (2009) Midwife struck off. 7 March.

Medicines and Healthcare products Regulatory Agency (MHRA) (2008) *Public Consultation (MLX 346): Proposals for amendments to the range of medicines which can be sold, supplied or administered by registered midwives.* London: MHRA.

National Patient Safety Agency (2009) *Annual Report and Accounts 08/09.* London: NPSA.

National Prescribing Centre (2004) *Patient Group Directions: A practical guide and framework of competencies for all professionals using patient group directions.* London: NPC.

National Society for the Prevention of Cruelty to Children (NSPCC) (2009) *Child Protection Register Statistics.* London: NSPCC.

National Statistics (2008) *NHS Workforce Census.* London: National Statistics.

Nazroo, J (2001) *Ethnicity, Class and Health.* London: Policy Studies Institute.

NHS Business Services Authority (NHSBSA) (2009) Midwife supervisor sentenced for £63,000 timesheet fraud. *NHSBSA News*, 24 June.

NHS Information Authority (NHSIA) (2002) *Share with Care!: People's views on consent and confidentiality of patient information.* London: NHSIA.

NHS Litigation Authority (NHSLA) (2009) *Annual Report and Accounts 2009.* London: NHSLA.

Northern Echo (2006) Staff looked at Sir Bobby's records, 25 November, p12.

Nursing and Midwifery Council (NMC) (2004a) *Code of Professional Conduct: Standards for conduct, performance and ethics.* London: NMC.

Nursing and Midwifery Council (NMC) (2004b) *Midwives Rules and Standards.* London: NMC.

Nursing and Midwifery Council (NMC) (2004c) *Complaints about Unfitness to Practise: A guide for members of the public.* London: NMC.

Nursing and Midwifery Council (NMC) (2006) *Standards of Proficiency for Nurse and Midwife Prescribers.* London: NMC.

Nursing and Midwifery Council (NMC) (2007) *NMC Advice Sheet on Record Keeping.* London: NMC.

Nursing and Midwifery Council (NMC) (2008a) *The Code: Standards of conduct, performance and ethics for nurses and midwives.* London: NMC.

Nursing and Midwifery Council (NMC) (2008b) *NMC Advice Sheet on Free Birthing.* London: NMC.

Nursing and Midwifery Council (NMC) (2008c) *Standards for Medicines Management.* London: NMC.

Nursing and Midwifery Council (NMC) (2009a) *Fitness to Practise Annual Report 2008-09.* London: NMC.

Nursing and Midwifery Council (NMC) (2009b) Supply and/or administration of medicine by student nurses and student midwives in relation to Patient Group Directions (PGDs) (NMC Circular 05/2009). London: NMC.

Nursing and Midwifery Council (NMC) (2009c) *Guidance on Professional Conduct for Nursing and Midwifery Students.* London: NMC.

Nursing and Midwifery Council (NMC) (2009d) *Record Keeping: Guidance for nurses and midwives.* London: NMC.

Nursing and Midwifery Council (NMC) (2009e) *Standards for Pre-registration Midwifery Education.* London: NMC.

Nursing and Midwifery Council (NMC) (2009f) *Fitness to Practise Annual Report: 1 April 2008 to 31 March 2009.* London: NMC.

Nursing and Midwifery Council (NMC) (2010a) Midwife struck off the register (Conduct and Competence Panel press release), 25 January.

Nursing and Midwifery Council (NMC) (2010b) *Update for Midwives.* London: NMC.

Office of National Statistics (ONS) (2009) *Live Births 2008*. London: The Stationery Office.

Payne, S (2004) Black nurse told not to treat white baby awarded £20,000. *The Daily Telegraph*, 18 May, p11.

Peterborough Today: The Evening Telegraph (2008) Hoodie yob attacks midwife on call. 13 February.

Prescott, A (2002) Childhood sexual abuse and the potential impact on maternity. *Midwifery Matters*, 92: 17–18.

Rideout, RW (1983) *Principles of Labour Law*. London: Sweet and Maxwell.

Royal College of Midwives (RCM) (2005) *Child Protection is Everybody's Business*. Available online at www.rcm.org.uk/midwives/news/rcm-in-the-news/child-protection-is-everybodys-business (accessed 1 June 2010).

Salmon, D, Baird, K, Price, S and Murphy, S (2004) *An Evaluation of the Bristol Pregnancy and Domestic Violence Programme*. Bristol: University of the West of England.

Savill, R (2005) Bodies in attic woman is spared jail. *Daily Telegraph*, 4 October, p13.

Stamford Mercury (2007) Sacked midwife free to practise again, 2 November, p3.

Taket, A (2004) *Tackling Domestic Violence: The role of health professionals*, 2nd edn. London: Home Office.

Thompson, I, Melia, K and Boyd, K (2000) *Nursing Ethics*. London: Churchill Livingstone.

UNICEF (2003) *A League Table of Child Maltreatment Deaths in Rich Nations* (Innocenti Report Card No. 5). Florence: UNICEF.

United Nations (UN) (1989) *Convention on the Rights of the Child* (adopted under General Assembly resolution 44/25). New York: United Nations.

Watson, R (2004) Woman who refused Caesarean charged with baby's murder. *The Times*, 13 March, p23.

Watson-Smyth, K (1997) Surrogate mother sets for legal battle. *Independent*, 3 November, p12.

Welsh Assembly Government (2000) *In Safe Hands: Implementing adult protection procedures in Wales*. Cardiff: Welsh Assembly Government.

Wheeler, R (2006) Gillick or Fraser? A plea for consistency over competence in children. *British Medical Journal*, 332: 807.

Williams, R (2009) Equality bill takes aim at 'institutional ageism' in NHS. *The Guardian*, 23 October, p12.

World Health Organisation (WHO) (2008) *Female Genital Mutilation* (Fact sheet 241). Geneva: WHO.

Index